Connected

a paradigm shift in how we view health

Andi Lew

National Library of Australia
Cataloguing-in-Publication Entry

ISBN
978-0-6484584-1-8 (paperback)
978-0-6484584-2-5 (ebook)

Health–Popular works.
Medicine, Popular.

Authors/Contributors:
Lew, Andi.

Cover and text design by Raspberry Creative
Layout and design by Busybird Publishing
Cover photography by Giorgia Maselli
Cover dress by Jason Grech Couture
Internals photography by Carlin Sterritt

Disclaimer:

Contents

Contents

Acknowledgements

Let's show gratitude for the bittersweet Global Destruction COVID-19 was. The Pandemic may also.be referred to as The Great Awakening. Through the terrible times, some have said that there was a silver lining they found and that they saw things differently now, with 2020 vision. My gift was clarity in my calling, which was my overwhelming responsibility to continue to help educate and inspire others towards optimal health naturally.

I would like to acknowledge the thousands of people that I have taught and /or seen professionally, for it is you and your results or your thirst for knowledge that drives me to continue teaching. To all the chiropractors, kinesiologists, medical doctors, natural health practitioners, trainers, authors, speakers, media, friends and family, thank you for your lessons, care and support.

Thank you to couture dress designer, Jason Grech and Giorgia Maselli, photographer, for making this vitalistic cover possible. Thank you to Carlin Sterritt for the internals photography.

I'd like to also acknowledge my ten year old son; Beaudy. He is an oracle and where I learn incredible insight. It is his insight that drove me to write the book. Our children are the future and we must listen to them whilst we are teaching them.

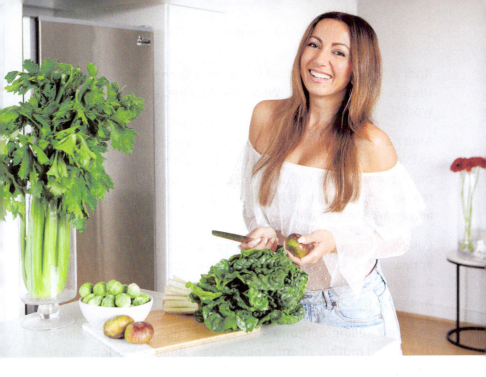

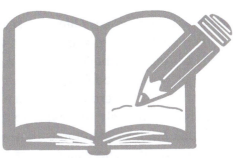

About the Author

Vivacious and effervescent; Andi Lew's radiant energy is often described as contagious. Australia's Herald Sun journalist Glenn Mitchell described her as 'naturally up', when he interviewed her about her first major role in Australian television as host on Channel 9's national dating television show, *Shopping for Love*. However, she is widely known for her work in wellness.

Andi is 47, but is often told she looks fifteen years younger and there's a reason for it. What she teaches is wellness; and it works!

Andi has taught millions through every media platform on how to live a healthier life naturally and now it's time to put it all in one book with this eighth title being the most asked for by her readers who begged to be informed how to stay well, youthful and energetic, naturally.

Celebrity manager Max Markson asked Andi to host the appearances of Arnold Schwarzenegger in Melbourne, Australia, and described her by saying, "Wellness is Andi's life work and passion."

This best-selling author, certified food, lifestyle and wellness coach, and mother of gorgeous 'tween' Beaudy has inspired so many with her lifestyle choices.

Andi has not always had an easy life, but keeps rising above the adversity and challenges to show others what is possible in life and health. Andi was bullied at school, pinned to the ground and called "Health Food Freak!" whilst the contents of her lunch were being smothered on her face. Andi distinctly remembers it. She was brought up always to eat well and was never allowed junk food, so the grapes that were pressed on her as she writhed on the cold concrete was always going to leave an imprint. Now, she looks back on it differently, as she is the last one laughing, but health isn't just about eating well, as you will soon learn.

After having appeared all over Australian and American live-television shows in press tours, the content from her seven health, parenting, nutrition and dating titles, has been valuable to viewers. As a well-respected and renowned "Wellness Expert", Andi decided to release Connected, a paradigm shift in how we view heath, her 8th book. It came about because of what she observed during the COVID-19 pandemic, a type of "biological warfare", or a "war on health" was how she described it. "I totally saw a divided globe," she said. "Those who wanted to place their health in someone else's hands and wait for magic cures, and those who took all the responsibility to look after their own wellness and rely on natural remedies and trust in their body's innate healing powers. I immediately went on a journey to heal the divide. We always need both."

As an observer of social culture, Andi is one to write about what she sees the world needs and her work often takes on a type of wellness crusade. This book is just that; connecting you, the reader to yourself and to your community and the earth because her calling, she believes, is to "love, serve, nurture", and it is through stories that we heal. "It is through fun that we learn," she said and believes her work is always both.

Often asked where her energy and youth come from, Andi loves to share her vitality secrets. Prior to a career in presenting, and as a wellness expert and coach, she had been a professional dancer and dance teacher. However, Andi was plagued with painful sciatica, a condition which affects the sciatic nerve, the longest nerve in the human body, causing pain and tingling in the leg and fainting attacks that prevented her from performing. It was only after years of struggle with these hidden health challenges that she was inspired to embark on a journey towards optimal health. The personal journey that followed led her to a new career path in health and wellness education and television.

She discovered the natural secrets to improving health and wellness when all other avenues failed, and these secrets improved both her quality of life and even her appearance. Andi is a qualified chiropractic assistant, has worked with some of the best in the profession for over 20 years, and has been asked to speak and to inspire at national seminars and at the New Zealand College of Chiropractic.

She won an award from the Chiropractor's Association of Australia for her dedication to the profession in 2009 in public education. To this day, nobody that isn't a chiropractor has won an award such as this. Andi's personal journey is so powerful, and her experiences so moving, that she has been written about in national magazines, podcasts and television interviews. Her clients have described her as truly inspirational.

As a woman of wide experience, education and natural nurturing instinct, Andi walks her talk and feels compelled to share her story so that others may benefit from what has made such a difference in her own life. The journey that led her to a greater quality of life by "accident", "health challenges" and "trauma" is illuminating and life-transforming. She constantly turns challenges, change and pain into growth and wellness.

Dedication

This book is for you, because we are mere reflections of each other. We are all the same; energy. What unifies us is diversity. There's unity in diversity, yet we all want the same things: to love and be loved. These simple birthrights are what help us navigate our health choices and lifestyle. You have chosen this book because you want more from your life and for your life.

This may be the first book of mine you have ever read, or your eighth, and every client or reader I have ever had the pleasure of inspiring, is what keeps me going. Your feedback on how I changed and shaped your life is heart-warming.

It is for the chiropractors and the allied and natural health profession that showed me the way and cared for me with their heart, hands and minds.

It is for all the people on the planet who are now finally ready to learn more about what true health, radiance and vitality is and where it comes from.

Most books are dedicated to others which is why I acknowledge only you. We are not separate. We are all mirrors of each other. We are all connected.

I also dedicate this book to myself. Through my own pain, I found the gifts. I keep looking for the lessons and light as we go inward and connect with our innate intelligence which is run by the universal intelligence. It is my calling to provide true health education and I am proud of myself for never giving up on constant wellness and evolution. I reflect that when you find your inspired destiny, and you have the courage to live it out, is when you are truly well. I wish to give you the same courage to set your heart on fire and continue to lead with love.

Through this holistic and healthy mindset and lifestyle is where your immune system may be boosted, and slowing of ageing begins.

Health begins with connection. Let's truly connect now. It's time for transformation through connection.

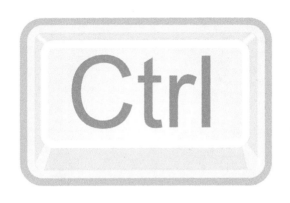

WELLNESS VS ALLOPATHY

CTRL + ALT + DEL
What You Know About Health.
Wellness is a Paradigm Shift.

*The Doctor of the future
will give no medicine; rather he
will educate his patients in the
care of the human frame, in diet and
in the prevention of disease.*

Thomas Edison

Lets begin with understanding the two models of care: wellness and allopathy. Wellness is about prevention and quality of life. The medical model which is allopathy, is about cure and early detection. They're two very different things when it comes to health languages. Health care is about maintaining the health you already have, but with wellness, there's no ceiling as to how well you can be.

Now, let's look at the notion that ageing well is the by-product of being well. How does one stay well in a modern world? We have much better sanitation and medicines, yet we are consuming more toxins or being surrounded by toxic stressors more than ever before.

You will discover why I have managed to slow ageing naturally, despite the setbacks I have had with various physical and mental health challenges. Good health isn't just luck or genes. We all have a genetic predisposition to certain illnesses, but these genes only get expressed in the right or "wrong" environment.

Slowing ageing and living a greater quality of life, needs to be the by-product of wellness.

I will teach you how to age well or slow ageing as a result of being well from the inside out. However, this is wellness which

Andi Lew

you may not have previously known and it's how I live my life. Where possible, I ascribe to a theory that a natural approach to health and always a holistic one. Nonetheless, there has been a divide and confusion amongst health practices. To be truly healthy begins with a paradigm shift in how you view health.

There's "well care" and there's "sick care", and they sometimes both get called "health care", but being healthy takes on all forms. What works for some doesn't work for others, and there's no "one size fits all" approach or formula when it comes to health.

The growing demand for natural health alternatives is being confused with the western medical model that treat and prescribe drugs. Both are different, and mean so well and both work, but for different reasons. This book aims to heal the divide because we do need both.

Let's look at labels and language. It is not "alternative" healthcare, because what is it an alternative to? We really do need both, and therefore I would like to suggest it be referred to as "complimentary". Labels create divide. We need to be mindful of our choice of words because we need unity and reconnection in order to be really well because you all discover that we are all connected.

Getting reconnected acknowledges that there is a movement of people who simply choose not to inject or ingest anything toxic. You will discover the reasons for this because toxicities disconnect brain to body and impact our overall health since toxins affect the nervous system and our gut health which is the second brain. It then in turn affects our hormones.

There's a myriad of non-invasive and natural ways to heal and stay well and the wellness revolution is in full swing.

There's a place for western medicine and one could never deny how far it has come in times of emergency. However, when we use drugs and medication on a regular basis, we can compromise our overall wellness or wellbeing. This toxic load and myriad of side effects get you on a drug merry-go-round, but the long-term goals you need to have is not to rely on medication to be well.

Let's refer to the quote at the beginning of this chapter.

The Doctor of the future will give no medicine; rather he will educate his patients in the care of the human frame, in diet and in the prevention of disease.

Thomas Edison

What the inventor Thomas Edison referred to in 1903 as a "doctor of the future" is so profound and even more relevant today than ever. Hippocrates, the father of medicine, said, "Natural forces within us are the true healers of disease."

You will soon discover the power of your body and how it has the ability to heal. When we work with the body instead of against its innate workings to heal, we give it the full opportunity to function at an optimal level.

The wellness model is a proactive approach. Then there is the allopathic model which is a reactive approach. It's called "allopathy", which is the medical model, and it is practiced with the approach of "waiting 'til it's broke to fix it".

The allopathic model has advanced so much. We now have the very best drugs, doctors and surgeons in the world. They have literally saved lives, yet we still have high rates of illness and disease.

Let's address the confusion with the allopathic model and what it is about. We rely on it to make us well, but it isn't about "wellness" or being proactive. There's a level of prevention but it is actually more like early detection. It's a model designed to get you back to where you began before you fell ill.

With wellness, there's no ceiling as to how healthy you can be and a healthy body looks different on every person. You might be fit, or lean, but it doesn't necessarily mean you are well.

The World Health Organisation even states in its definition of health, that "Health is a state of complete physical, mental and social wellbeing, and not merely the absence of disease infirmity."

Wellness is a change of perception and a shift in paradigms on how you view health and your symptoms. Being really well is the state of optimal function on every level.

There's nobody to blame though. We just haven't really understood our health up until recently, and it took a pandemic for the world to want to understand and learn more about our health.

Why do some get sick and others are asymptomatic? What makes someone more well or resilient than another? Perhaps the quality of your life is dependent on the quality of questions you ask. High-quality questions create the opportunity for a high-quality life.

Our bodies are an incredible thing. The more we ask, the more we learn, and even then, the more we know, the more we realise we don't know. There is so much to learn about our intricately designed bodies.

The very basic information on how our bodies work to heal and to cleanse is what I'm going to empower you with, including how you can support it so that at least then you are able to make more informed decisions for yourself. I would like for you to let your choices come from a place of inspiration and that you also start taking full responsibility of your own health.

Please know that these steps to radiant wellness are not hidden. They also can add to how well we age. For some years though, these steps have been available to anyone motivated and diligent enough to search them out, but they were like the scattered pieces of a puzzle. Not until now have they all been brought together to reveal the total picture of what true health is, and how to achieve and maintain it. The concept of real wellness contradicts much of what we have been led to believe for so long.

The by-product of being really well is "ageing less", or at least "ageing well". So why haven't we used wellness more to help how we age? Why do we rely on a magic cream, cure or procedure? It's all about to change when you understand how we viewed health before and how we want to view it now.

We would go to our doctor when we are sick, but where do we go when we're "well"? Wait, what? – see a health professional when you're well? I know the notion may sound odd, but it's actually very wise because it's so much easier to stay well than to get well, right? We have been so conditioned to work ever longer and harder, to ignore warning signs and symptoms, and to suffer in silence, or to take a pill and soldier on. So have we forgotten what health really is?

More and more people at ever-younger ages have become reliant on often unnecessary drugs. The false belief that illness is a natural and unavoidable state for human beings has become an unquestioned truth, fostered by a multibillion-dollar industry which has controlled the mainstream health profession for decades by "selling sickness".

Despite the proliferation of new and powerful drugs on the market, diseases such as cancer and heart disease grow more prevalent with each passing year, obesity is fast becoming the number-one health risk in the modern world, and depression and other psychological imbalances are afflicting more people than ever before. We are starting to understand how living in isolation where the lack of touch, human connection, support, resources, and basic nutrition all contribute to our overall mental and physical wellbeing.

No matter how advanced medicine becomes, sometimes waiting for symptoms to appear before reacting is just too late. The chemical- and surgical-intervention movements have had a good long run, but they just haven't always delivered what we all hoped and believed they could give us health.

Since the dawn of the new millennium, *wellness* has itself become a new multibillion-dollar industry. You only need to look at the millions of people who attend wellness summits, Natural Products Expos in Anaheim like Expo West and their other event called Expo East, many more who study natural professions, and the millions searching for new wellness products and platforms. The old ways have fallen short of their promise, and the increasing collective of literally billions of people are now exploring the above, buying books on healing and searching the internet for natural solutions for living.

The pendulum has swung for so long towards surgery and drugs, and now it is inevitably swinging just as hard the other way – towards wellness. Rather than merely being healed of illnesses, people want more for their health; they are sick and tired of being sick and tired.

In response to this tidal wave of social awareness toward vitality and self-determination, the business culture has made changes that would have been unthinkable in the past:

- Weight-loss is a multibillion-dollar industry, with gyms, diets, personal fitness trainers, books, videos and online programs, calorie-control centres, exercise and nutrition podcasts or streaming shows.

- Nutritional companies and food manufacturers are going "plant based", "vegan", "organic", "SLS and paraben free", "gluten free", "NO additives", "refined sugar free", "FODMAP friendly" and "preservative free".

- International fast food chains have added "healthy" options on their menus in a bid to keep up with our demands.

- Proliferating "lifestyle" businesses and magazines promote quality of life.

- Workplace occupational health and safety officers are being appointed within companies to monitor conditions of employment.

- Organisations invested in yoga or meditation rooms for their employees as the link between health and productivity became common knowledge.

- Employers offered wellness perks to their staff with company sponsored massages, treatments or seminars.

- Caffeine alternatives like matcha, turmeric, cacao and beetroot lattes are now on the menu.

- Multinational companies offered employees incentives for healthy, *preventative* lifestyles.

- Since the year 2000, we moved away from milk and as we started consuming dairy alternatives like soy, and it continued into a myriad of other healthier options. Now we are becoming more mindful with our eating choices and consuming less meat or no animal products as we care for the environment, look after our health or make a heart choice.

- The demand for wellness and prevention is so great that even pharmaceutical companies are selling vitamins and supplements, or promoting wellness and mindfulness.

- Chiropractors like Dr Fabricio Mancini, author of *Chicken Soup for the Chiropractic Soul*, and other leaders in the over 100-year-old profession lead this return to wellness origins. Chiropractors are getting amazing results for conditions other than just headaches or pack pain.

Our appetite for organics is growing and with interest in the quality of soil, we are looking towards biodynamic and regenerative farming.

In "well care", I have known some no longer use the word "patient" as it refers to "one who suffers". Changing this label has changed the whole perspective on sickness versus wellness.

It appears the western world has decided that simply not having symptoms just isn't good enough anymore. We have collectively created a worldwide wellness revolution through our demand for *true* health. So, if you are tired of the drug merry-go-round with all its side effects, and if you would love to have youth and vitality without intervention, then this book is for you.

The Secret: Prevention IS the Cure

There is a revolution taking place and you are part of it. The questioning of medical authorities has arisen because not only are more people becoming sicker, but healthcare costs are rising beyond the ability of most individuals and even governments to pay.

The physical, social and financial costs are just too high, and spiralling further out of control. Wouldn't it be wonderful to live in a world where we invested in prevention and education and actually saved the government money in sick care? My aim is to keep you well. Investing in your health is the only thing that can guarantee a return in this current economic climate. The current generation wants to take back control of their own health.

So, it's time to apply the following wellness principles in order that glowing health can be achieved easily and without side effects. As an added bonus to creating "optimal health", you may boost your immune system, decrease the effects of ageing and take years off your appearance.

Ageing is much more of a choice than people ever dream. One of modern medicine's great breakthroughs is a realisation that the body is not an object, but a process with no preordained limits.

Deepak Chopra

So why do so many rely so much on medication and why do professionals *forget* to tell us how to achieve optimal health? What is it that gives top athletes, business people, and entertainers the vital edge? What are the healthiest people on the planet doing?

I have liaised with many of the most inspired and informed people on earth over my 28 years of being in wellness, and the time has come to share with you some of the world's best-kept health secrets. This book reveals information on the whole spectrum of health, including chiropractic and nervous system health, assimilation of nutrition, and how taking medication and consuming diet drinks might be compromising your overall wellbeing and healing capacity! It will inspire your health and wellness ideas and may challenge some old beliefs.

You are about to discover what top athletes, television stars, and countless other leaders have all used to achieve excellence in their chosen fields. You see, we don't need any more studies to show that exercise benefits you or to prove that fresh food is better than packaged food. What we need is to understand that our health choices bear consequences that are either positive or negative.

We have so much to gain from embracing this wellness revolution – knowledge, empowerment and a better quality of life for our children, and their children. There are already millions of doctors beginning to work in partnership with allied health professionals like chiropractors, personal trainers, and a host of natural health carers. They have been inspired to question their assumptions, to look into the power of vitamins and nutrition, and to keep up-to-date with research into the latest drugs and their side effects. The old ways are changing, the new way is here.

What's "true wellness"?

Health and healing is a deep subject that will never truly end, but this book is distilled into the key things that will have the most profound and immediate effect on your life today, if you *apply* them. You will also start to understand that the way your body responds to stressors is actually a healthy adaptation for survival and if we understand it and work with it, then we will notice it is a "wellness response" to an external threat or an internal struggle. I call this the "wellness response" because how your body adapts and is designed to heal is incredible.

We need to give the body the right environment though. There are, of course, limitations of matter, but there are always things you can do to at least improve the quality of your life or stop things worsening and sometimes even improve or heal. Working with the body and allowing it to flourish and thrive is the "next level" or "true" wellness.

We will address the cumulative effects of lifestyle choices and the four toxic stressors that impact to be truly well.

You will understand the innate wisdom of the body, how your nerve system works, intelligent nutrition, the dangers of drug side effects, the quality of your water and hydration, the power of your own mind to create disease or wellness within your body and much more. You cannot read this material without having a radical shift in health consciousness and in the quality of your life. It will encourage you to have a better relationship with yourself, and with those whom you trust to care for your health as you learn to ask better questions.

When we share these secrets, there is a wide range of responses. Some people are surprised that there are only these few chapters and steps. They are usually the ones who are already proactive in their healthcare, with a good relationship with their doctor or alternative practitioner, while a few don't have a need to see a doctor at all and they have accessed true wellness now.

Some feel shocked, confused or even betrayed that this information was withheld because so much vital knowledge is available to them now – these are the people with the most to gain, whose lives will be most transformed by it.

Remember though, don't blame your doctor for not telling you about the keys to wellness. It's just a paradigm shift in thinking and the way they have been taught health is to operate or medicate. This is their area of expertise. Be patient with them. Many don't yet know this themselves and may be learning right along with you.

Others also may just not be ready to learn about how to take back control of our own health, because it means not just a shift in your thinking but also you will need to be responsible for your own health instead of not doing anything to improve on it daily.

I too have not always been ready to heal. Any time is a good time to start and any little part you can do adds up. Our souls are only able to process so much at one time. We can't force healing. We need breaks and to wait for life to happen in between. Just enjoy the journey though because with wellness there is no destination. There's no ceiling nor end point, because you can never be too well. During my own pain and life challenges, as we all have them, I soon realised two things: my responsibility and the familiarity.

You see, I have been teaching and writing or presenting wellness for 28 years and I was and am powerfully inspiring because I walk my talk. Unfortunately, the second thing was that I realised I had felt pain like this before, and it was time to pattern break. This information is crucial because emotional trauma can lead to ill health and is a huge part of wellness.

Your emotional stressors may not be like mine, but any stress, trauma and lack of support can manifest into actual physical illness if not dealt with. I was living a very healthy life, eating well, using natural healing modalities, avoiding toxins, exercising and the like. The one thing that was really missing from my health, was the emotional, but you may need the physical or the connection of all the following modalities to really fly now. I am hoping it inspires you to do the same as I continue to do, year after year, commit to wellness, and address some things you may not have had the courage to commit to before. It would be physical, chemical, nutritional, emotional, financial or spiritual areas. It may even be an environmental toxic stress. Some of our trauma is even generational.

Whatever we have been dealt with is up to us to heal. It even took a pandemic for us to realise that we had been triggered by our past traumas and it was finally time to heal those too. We soon learned the we can no longer sit back and cruise because how we view health is never going to be the same again.

I had tried to address the entire spectrum of my traumas over the years but this time, as my health was in my hands, drenched in tears, and held in the embrace of my friend's arms, I looked up. I literally changed my physiology and looked up as a thought of clarity came to mind. Please note that the change in physiology changes the chemistry and in turn the emotional status. What if this was all a lesson? What could I learn from this?

Have you ever felt this way when something terrible happens and you wonder, "Why me?" I began to sit with the journey and you will soon learn why this is helpful when wanting to achieve true health and connection. With this acceptance, I gave myself actual permission to take time out and truly reconnect again to heal. Maybe the whole of 2020 was forced upon us all to do just that?

I usually never stop. I am wired and inspired, because I do what I love. Do you ever find yourself constantly thinking you really need to stop and look at something on a much deeper level? What might be holding us all back from optimal heath? We don't need to be a victim of our genes and past family illnesses if we can radically change lifestyle. You will learn more about this and epigenetics in the following pages. Changing signals from brain to body is where we can start to change DNA function and expression. We will always have a genetic predisposition, but genes only express themselves when we give them the right (or wrong) environment.

My attitude of forgiving, acknowledging, being present and having unconditional love for myself was one of the reasons I stayed so young and well. I noted that I needed to be doing this now, more than ever. What if our thoughts were the very thing that makes us sick or well? If a thought could make you sick, surely it can make you well too.

I understand that you may not have the time to research the huge spectrum of the latest health breakthroughs, which is why I've done it for you, step by step and chapter by chapter. *Connected to Wellness* is not only my life's work and passion, but also a summary and extension of most of my books.

I aim to not only educate, empower and inspire you, but also help save you a lot of time and money, and maybe even extend the quality of your life with this book. The best part is, your health and vitality are about putting the power back in your hands. From now on, it's up to you. I'm with you on this radiant wellness journey that will take you to the next level.

References

Articles

World Health Organisation, https://www.who.int/about/who-we-are/constitution

A Risk Assessment of Cervical Manipulation Vs NSAIDs for the Treatment of Neck Pain

Dabbs V, DC and Lauretti WJ, DC. JMPT 1995; 18(8):530–6

Australian Organics 2019 Market record, https://austorganic.com/publications/ao-market-report-2019/

Books

Dr Bruce Lipton, *The Biology of Belief*, Hay House Inc

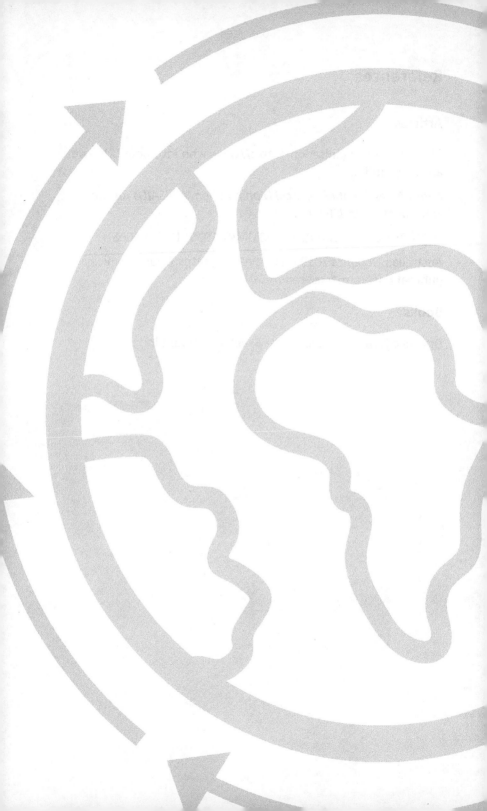

1

EVERYTHING IS CONNECTED

Human Connection,
Connecting to Our Body,
and Our Planet is Where
We Find Wellness.

All great truth passes through three stages:
First, it is ridiculed.
Second, it is violently opposed.
Third, it is accepted as being self-evident.

Arthur Schopenhauer
Philosopher (1788–1860)

Can you imagine if one day you were walking along a beautiful mountainous landscape that hugged a river bed, and you were taking in the absolute serenity and magnitude of beauty, but a vision of panic at the foot of the river disturbed you? You witness an exasperated man who's kneeling near the water, scooping up dead fish and resuscitating or rescuing them and then throwing them back into the water. You're standing there watching in awe and panic because there's that many dying and they're flowing down the stream.

The man looks up at you after feeling your presence and says, "Don't just stand there! Get help! I need help! Can't you see I am saving lives here and you should be down here helping me!"

As much as you know that he is right and a surge of cortisol rushes through your body, which is the hormone designed to make you move fast and take action as a stress response, you also immediately hear your inner self questioning why so many fish are dying in the first place. You don't take the man's anger and frustration personally because he is well intentioned. He indeed is saving lives. You decide, however, to make your way to the top of the river and discover just why these fish are falling ill in the first place.

This is ADDRESSING THE CAUSE, NOT JUST THE SYMPTOMS.

However, the natural health profession has been challenged within the western world, just as much as it has been supported.

Whilst both approaches are needed, the bottom of the river is where the emergency care lies. The top is where disease began. It is the state of disease and dysfunction you're looking to improve because you don't want to wait until there's panic and a rescue operation needed. More lives can be saved up top, at the beginning, at the state of disease, and not to wait until you get to a state of disease. This is a wellness approach and it is holistic. It recognises that everything is connected and when we disrupt the balance, we can create illness and disharmony. The disharmony analogy can be used for our bodies or the earth itself. In fact, we are all connected.

What if everything is connected, and once we take care of our health with this notion in mind, we in turn, also take care of the planet? What if who we are, how we heal ourselves and our relationships to everything is the answer to better health? This respect for all life and living things is going to help you to work with our body and want more for yourself and your environment.

Social distancing caused a disconnect with each other and an increase in social media networking.

It was the perfect breeding ground for either propaganda to be taught or truth to be told. People searched for science. The process of science is designed to challenge ideas through research, and in this thirst for knowledge, we discover a 'back and forth' of how things work. I started questioning whether the only true science could be noted as quantum physics, where some things may be hard to see or feel, yet still exist, and an equal and opposite energy of both sides are always going to be present, which represents perfect balance. I would like to suggest that both propaganda and truth were both present during 2020.

As we disconnected from Mother Earth though, we further disconnected to ourselves and the way our bodies are designed to heal.

Dr Zach Bush, MD, said, "Not so long ago, the world was rich with microbial life. Plants and animals flourished. The air was clean, the water was pure and humans thrived. The next level of connection will demand the evolution of all of us. That's because we are deeply connected with nature."

I wrote in my sixth book, *Wellness Loading – Disconnect to Reconnect*:

> *The key to being really well is to stay connected to all areas of your life. Connectors show you how to detox not just your body but also your mind and spirit. Learn how to just "be", tune in and connect with food and nature again, for an overall much needed detox in the digital era. As cliché as it sounds, it's really all about balance.*

Our First People in Australia talk about 'connection to Country' all the time.

Did you know that we are made up of 70–80% water? If you knew that, then did you know that plants too are made up of the same percentage of water and so too is the earth? Can you see the connection to all living things?

We need to acknowledge this connection and understand that taking a pill will disconnect your actual self from brain to body as it sends distorted messages from brain to body. This is effective for a short-term solution in response to an emergency, but if this is applied over time, then it will keep us disconnected to mother earth too. As a result, our decision-making won't be as mindful.

Whilst painkillers and some drugs are needed in emergency situations, let's remember that we need to stay connected to our bodies and find ways to detox, cleanse and heal naturally by getting more connected on a day-to-day basis.

If you already rely on medication, and have a condition, then you might want to find ways to work with your health practitioner to help you on this journey. Sometimes, there are limitations of matter, but other times there might be something else that you could explore that will improve the quality of your life. However, what you decide is yours. It's your choice and your life. This is your body and you get to choose how you want to live your life.

To feel is to heal. Just like when we strain our ankle, the pain is there to remind us to not put so much pressure on it. The body has an innate intelligence and way of assisting. We are designed to heal through the workings of our nervous system, which you will discover are about soon, and we are wired to connect.

You could also use this analogy of the healing ankle with our hearts and minds. When we suffer emotional trauma or a broken heart, it can be very painful. You only have to look at the Shakespeare's play of *Romeo & Juliet* to understand how love, perception and loss can turn to ill health.

Sometimes, some of us have relied on anti-depressants to get us through a period of pain, but when we're finally ready to address the cause, we need a huge heart. This is where we will need the courage to show up and be seen with all our pain and vulnerability. We need more connection, more compassion and the word "courage" actually comes from the French word "le couer" which means "the heart".

So we need to be whole hearted to feel and heal through a divine discomfort. This is where growth lies. Otherwise, we end up numbing our feelings through addiction to a disconnector. Know that when you are in a state of loss and extreme emotion, you're not necessarily "down", maybe you are just having "downtime".

We all have it and we all need it. It is healthy to stop and feel, or stop and heal, and you can choose to call this a "rebalance". This slowing down gives us time to reflect, find support or just "be" instead of "do". We are so busy that we forget to be present.

Gone are the times where we are being brought up in a society when "children should be seen but not heard", or "men should not cry", and this is something that has been taught through years of generational trauma. It is up to us to break the pattern. For example, did you know that sad tears have analgesic properties? This is why sometimes when you have a good cry, you might feel so much better afterwards.

If you are always down and have been diagnosed with depression or anxiety and disorders such as PTSD, remember to be gentle on yourself and understand it might take more time, but you can continue or just begin the journey of healing and work together with your choice of professionals to do the work. Get reconnected to your heart.

Getting connected to your heart can help not only you, but the world around you, for we are all connected. We are mirrors of each other.

Healthy connection and reconnection will allow you to start listening to your body and giving it what it needs. How many times have we been programmed with pharmaceutical ads to take a drug and "soldier on"? I remember working at a chiropractic practice and a person came in for care explaining she has been suffering from headaches. The chiropractor asked what type of headaches and she replied, "Oh, just the normal types of headache once a week." Do you see how she was conditioned to believe that a weekly headache is normal? Headaches are not normal and a drug doesn't address it, it only masks the symptom.

You see, for so long we were taught that when you have one part of you that is sick, you treat just that part. You have tonsillitis? Remove the tonsils. However, that fails to acknowledge that the tonsils are connected to other parts and just as we remove one animal from an ecosystem and disrupt the balance, if we do the same to the human body, then the same disruption occurs. We are incredibly adaptive though and our bodes can operate without limbs and organs but let's always work with the notion in mind that everything is connected and respect this not only in our bodies but with the earth too.

There's not merely one way to practice health and you will (as cliched as it sounds) find out what works best for you. Just like any journey there will be growth.

We often act a little invincible and neglect ourselves or the planet and leave our health in the hands of brilliant experts only to forget to actually take on board what it is we can be doing to make their job easier, or just become more well by taking action and committing to them.

Maturity means taking responsibility for yourself, which many find challenging. But because you will be changing the quality and quantity of your *life*, I assure you that the rewards will be well worth the effort. As a certified food, lifestyle and wellness coach who has practiced and managed wellness clinics for many years, I can tell you that the journey is easy only when you understand the "why". When you are empowered with knowledge on "why" you, then it becomes more inspiring to commit to.

Nobody should tell you that you should do anything. We are more empowered when we understand the benefits of a choice and not the fear of when we don't.

We are often only told what can benefit our health by informing us of what will go wrong if we don't do something that will benefit us. This act hasn't always worked. Imagine you were told of all the things you'd be given as a result of changing your lifestyle, like ageing less, boosting immunity or a better quality of life, as opposed to only seeing warning labels on boxes or be scared into what illness you might get if you don't do something recommended?

In order to begin, in order to go anywhere it's vital to know where you are now. The quick quiz below will give you a clear picture of where you are in terms of your overall physical health. And remember, the more honest you are, the more effective the test will be.

Remember, you might be fit or lean, but it does not necessarily mean you are well because a healthy body looks different on every person. We will also unlock in the coming pages what ageing well really means. Let's remove the stigma about what we once thought beauty is or was. You are about to learn a whole new level of attraction and it stems with wellness.

How Well Are You?

Is your diet generally:

A. filled with lots of alkalised, filtered and clean water, plants and live foods that are fresh and full of colour, mostly organic and often raw with limited packaged foods?

B. made up of that caffeine hit, average amounts of tap water, some fresh food, but conventional, with some packaged food for convenience?

C. made up of mostly take-away or packaged foods, with limited fresh produce? You forget to drink water at all, rely on stimulants like caffeine quite heavily, and mostly use a microwave to cook and/or rarely cook.

Is your week:

A. filled with lots of mindfulness, body movement or at least a minimum of three exercise sessions, and do you sit and sleep with good posture?

B. comprised of lots of disconnect in choices because of stress, unbalanced emotions, with a single exercise session? Do you try to have a good posture in spite of your difficult work conditions?

C. devoid of work/life balance, with a disconnect to your emotions or needing help in understanding them, no movement or exercise, and at best you only occasionally leave your desk to walk around a little, slouching when standing and slumping on the couch at home?

Are you the kind of person who:

A. maintains a positive outlook on life, has many friends or social support, laughs a lot and takes time to smell the roses?

B. is somewhat volatile emotionally, with a few positive friends but more with a negative or grudging outlook on the world?

C. is often moody, socially isolated, easily get upset or angry, with an unsupportive work environment or relationship?

When it comes to your health, do you:

A. have the attitude that prevention is better than cure and are very active in maintaining your health?

B. try to be proactive about your health and seek advice, but delay or avoid acting due to the many reasons/excuses that you create?

C. have an attitude of "If it ain't broke, don't fix it", and wait until you are so unwell that you must rely on medication to "cure" you?

Mostly A

If you circled mostly A, then you are likely to be the kind of person who is living a healthy life full of open-minded questions rather than closed assumptions. You tend not to accept the opinions of the mass media or mainstream media at face value, preferring to look deeper into areas that interest you and doing your own research.

You very rarely get sick, and when you do, you recover quite quickly without the need for drug intervention. You can't remember the last time you were unwell, or you remember it well as something which happened a long time ago and you recovered very quickly. You value your health very highly, and believe there is no price one can put on it.

You are living a great quality of life.

Mostly B

You circled mostly B? Well, you are enthusiastic about making healthy changes, but rarely do you have the time, energy or will to be as healthy as you'd like to be. It takes a lot of time to research and you have had to prioritise other things lately. You tend to give authority to others such as friends, family or doctors, and allow yourself to be influenced by them if you don't have the information to back up your health choices. You dedicate a reasonable amount of your resources to eating good foods and to prevention.

Your health is usually better than the "average" person.

Mostly C

Circling C takes real honesty and I admire your integrity. By the end of this book you will be inspired to greater health. As awareness is the first step, just by being committed enough to read it you are 50% there already.

If you are past your middle years, then your health may have been severely challenged. And if you are younger and make no changes, then it probably will be. You haven't given much thought or care to your health and wellbeing, and are usually preoccupied with other people or projects that are more important to you.

You tend to accept the health opinions of authority figures and rarely have the time to question or seek second opinions. You forget to listen to your body's signs and symptoms and switch them off with a drug or alcohol or any other stimulant or addiction, which you may not even be aware of, to block it out and keep soldiering on.

You are lovable. You are doing the best job you can with the resources and knowledge you have.

This health behaviour and lifestyle is all about to change for you.

What Optimal Health Is

The choices you make today affect your life tomorrow, but without knowledge you may not be aware of the end results of your choices. Having said that, whatever choice you make though is right for you and at the time of your life that you make that choice; is divinity in timing. This is because the life actually is about timing. We need to look at what's going on for you holistically. As a wellness coach, I always look at every little thing that is going on in your life, because we make choices based on how we feel we can survive all the other areas of our lives too; financial, emotional, spiritual, family and environmental too. Sometimes, people go so far as to looking into their past generational and planetary activity also. It is all connected.

Even with the general health awareness that exists today, most of us believe that it doesn't really apply to us, that we are somehow special and we'll be spared the consequences of our daily actions. The truth is, the body has its own laws and there is always a price to pay for ignoring them. It all eventually catches up. The body can only adapt for so long to the stressors. You are definitely special, that's why I care so much that I feel compelled to share these secrets of health with you, but it's time you began to treat yourself with the care you deserve. Why should I be keeping them all to myself? How can I be happy when others are sad, or at least living a life with less that optimal health?

In every area of life, there are consequences. Let's talk about what happens when we leave something too long before we address it. If you take your partner for granted, don't they let you know about it in no uncertain terms? If you are careless in your work, aren't there repercussions? If you ignore your finances for too long, isn't there an eventual accounting that can be both painful and humbling? We all know this, because we've *experienced* it, and yet, because of the sometimes decades-long lag between actions and their results, we imagine that somehow the area of health will be magically different. Isn't that a funny notion? Do you think it is because we rely on the advancement of medical technology and doctors because they're so good that we wait for them to save us? Leaving our health until it is too late isn't different to any of the other examples, and it requires as much attention, care and respect as any other area of your life.

So why has this healthy "wellness" way of living become the world's best-kept health secret? Why is it only now amongst a wellness revolution and global pandemic that we decide to discover how we can better our health and quality of life? It's because we have actually left this too long and it is finally time to start becoming a healthier human race and this in turn affects our planet. Because it is all so connected, remember?

> **Secret** /'si:krit adj. & n. _adj. 1. kept or meant to be kept private, unknown or hidden from all, or all but a few 2. acting or operating secretly 3. a mystery 4, a valid but not commonly known or recognised method of achieving or maintaining something.
>
> **Concise Oxford Dictionary**

It is time to no longer keep this information a secret or in private circles. It is the time to share it with the world so that we can all benefit.

In the past, we have blindly accepted that the friendly family doctor should be our first resort, and that they alone should bear the responsibility for our health education. They still can and do have a responsibility as a primary health practitioner, but we have unwisely used them as our primary *"sick care"* practitioner. We only go to doctors when we are sick, but this is a complete misunderstanding of the nature of health and care. In fact, achieving health isn't about waiting until you're sick to do something about it, or simply taking a pill.

Allopathy versus Wellness

Now, there isn't necessarily any moral corruption here. Many professionals and people are sincerely striving to alleviate human suffering, but their approach to wellness is based upon false premises. They are working from the "allopathic" model, a term created in the 19th century by Samuel Hahnemann to describe a medical system based upon treating illness by creating effects in the body that are opposite to the disease symptoms. It differs philosophically and practically from the "homeopathic" model (from *homeo*, meaning "the same"), which treats by mimicking symptoms and felt to be more humane by its practitioners – but both treat illness.

Allopathy is a mechanistic approach – that is, when we have a part in us that is broken or ill we take that part out and replace it, or cure it. For example, the mechanistic approach to tonsillitis (inflamed tonsils) would be to medicate or to remove the tonsils. This is just how medical workers are trained. So don't blame doctors or drug companies, they are skilful specialists in the allopathic model, which is based upon sick care. We need them when we are sick because we are all human and all of us at some point have left something too late, but it is time to make a change now and be more proactive and preventative.

Therefore, and this is the vital difference, the wellness model doesn't *treat* or *cure* anything. It is a proactive rather than a reactive approach. To use the previous example, the wellness approach would focus on *why* the tonsils are inflamed in the first place by addressing the cause and not just the symptom. In fact, the real wellness approach would not wait for the inflammation symptom to occur before looking at what could possibly create such an inflammation and thus develop strategies to avoid it in the first place.

Well care or wellness is about maintaining someone who is asymptomatic (healthy or symptom-free), or improving someone who wants even better health by helping their body to function at an even more effective level.

The opposite of mechanism is holism and it is at the core of the wellness philosophy. You may have heard of the "holistic approach", but not put too much thought into what it really means. I am a lover of language so let's break it down. Holism doesn't view human beings as a collection of unrelated parts, but respects that everything in the body and mind is subtly connected. There is no "robbing Peter to pay Paul" trade-off between treatment and side effects in holistic care.

All credit to those doctors who do have a holistic approach to health, and they are a growing body in the profession, but also keep in mind that they are still *curing symptoms or disease.* Whether you treat an illness with a chemical cocktail of drugs or a natural selection of homeopathy or vitamins, it is still a *treatment* for disease. The wellness model isn't a treatment. You don't have to be sick in order to get well!

Orthodox medicine is excellent, even unparalleled in treating acute or traumatic injuries and conditions, and we ignore it at our cost. However, we should be more concerned about the health choices we make in our lives on a daily basis *before* we need medical attention. In some cases, by the time we finally receive a diagnosis, it is too late to get well.

If a woman is wise enough to have her breasts examined, a lump can be found and removed. However, by the time any lump is large enough to be detected by a mammogram (breast cancer examination) that potential cancer will have been present and growing for at least six years! With foreknowledge, so much could have been done in those six years or more to keep the cells from ever reaching that condition. The mammogram is an excellent tool for diagnosing breast cancer, but it is only early detection, not prevention. There's a difference.

It is possible to be sick long before the body reveals any symptoms, like being unaware of tooth decay until it is well advanced. There may be no symptoms, but there is disfunction (impaired or less than optimal activity) which, if left for too long, may cause discomfort or become dis-ease (pain), and then eventually full-blown disease. Checking your body for disfunction is like checking to make sure your parachute is correctly packed *before* you jump out of the plane. True wellness requires us to be not just responsive, but proactive.

Medicine has become technically advanced, yet paradoxically we are getting unhealthier and sicker – medical statistics confirm ever-increasing rates of chronic disease and illness. At present, one in every three people will at some point in their life develop cancer. This is a shocking statistic in the face of so much technical skill, considering how many billions of dollars are spent on healthcare.

However, there is a small but growing minority of people who are avoiding this epidemic. This select group is participating in the wellness revolution, and they are reversing the normal trend by actually growing in health and vitality as they age. This is not merely a matter of luck and good genetics; whilst that certainly helps, genes only get expressed in the right or "wrong" environment. We certainly have a genetic predisposition to certain illnesses but we don't have to be a victim to it if we can learn more about epigenetics. This is what scientist Dr Bruce Lipton, PhD, talks about in his book *The Biology of Belief*. Surviving illness is also a direct result of the choices they are making on a daily basis.

Now, there is no question that modern medicine is extending our life span. In fact, over the past 100 years, life expectancy in the industrialised world has increased by 2 years per decade – that's 20%, or an extra 12 minutes each and every hour of your life.

But now the question is, what is the quality of those extended lives? People are living longer, but they are doing so with auto-immune diseases such as arthritis and rheumatism, with chronic pain requiring constant medication, with heart disease, cancer, Alzheimer's and Parkinson's, ADHD, autism, allergies, and a host of other maladies which greatly reduce their ability to enjoy that longer life.

As our lifespan lengthens and our capacity to accrue wealth increases, our expectations also rise. We have so many more options today, and it is no longer enough just to survive, we want to live. We want to retain our youth and health to a degree that was unthinkable in the past: women want to preserve their fertility as they choose to have babies later in life; those with fulfilling careers question compulsory retirement and want to continue to contribute their hard-won wisdom and experience; the retired don't want to just sit on the back porch complaining about their back and bladder problems, they want to be socially active, to dance and ski and cruise and travel the world, enjoying the rewards after a lifetime of work.

It is a cruel irony that with such extraordinary advances in science and medicine, so many people are unable to enjoy their hardearned rest because their bodies have simply ceased functioning due to a lifetime of neglect or misuse. The medical response to this situation has been to rely on a multitude of drugs to "manage" the various conditions, invasive surgery, chemotherapy or radiation therapy to remove or destroy damaged tissues, and cosmetic surgery and procedures to restore the superficial appearance of youth.

Now, I do not judge you if this is what you decide to do, but do know that youthful looks and ageing well is possible naturally?

Appearances have become more important than reality, and the reality is that true dynamic health isn't about aesthetic beauty or youth. It's not about your size or weight or age, or even the number of wrinkles on your face. No, true health is about the *functioning* of the marvellously complex and intricate miracle that is your body. I wonder when we will start to also find this level of wellness highly attractive? Wellness is about living your life in a way that will create a healthier you on a cellular level.

Our bodies are building and destroying cells in their billions, all day, every day. They are living factories, creating us anew each day, and they need quality materials to create quality cells. When you make healthier choices, your body's cell function and production flourishes, and so do *you*. If we want vitality and radiance in our lives, then we must understand that it's not really about the outside, but the inside – that it comes from a state of optimal inner health.

Radiant health is not an accident, it's about the choices you make that allow your body to function better on the inside. This is what I want for you. I am also a fan of removing the stigma of what is beauty and how we view ageing. When we empower ourselves with the knowledge of what we can do to be more well and action it, results will start to take shape and how you look may also change in a positive way. Beauty and agelessness will be the by-product of being really well.

The truth about real health though is, that it is not about how you look or feel; it's how you *function*, and it's a disturbing fact that in most instances you will be completely unaware that you are unwell.

How is this possible that we may not even know? You are about to grasp just how connected we really are. We function through our nerve system (the brain, spinal cord, and the nerves that branch off of it), and less than 10% of that system is dedicated to *feeling* nerves. Its main job is to facilitate the function of every organ, cell and tissue in the body, so that by the time you feel a symptom, the disfunction may have been around for a long time.

Symptoms are usually warning signs that some malfunction is well advanced – anti-tobacco lobbies use this to great effect. They show repulsive, graphic images on advertisements and warning labels, of toxic effluents squeezed out of the lungs of smokers or autopsies of diseased organs, illustrating very powerfully and effectively that we simply aren't aware of most of what is going on inside us until it's too late.

Children who become diagnosed with cancer is a perfect example of this. They may grow up like any other happy, playful child, with no hint that they are in any way unhealthy. Then one day a complaint of a tummy ache, which becomes more frequent over the following weeks, leading to a CT (Computed Tomography) scan at the hospital, and a massive abdominal tumour is revealed which the radiologist estimates had been there for about four years. Sadly, for half her life she had been desperately unhealthy, yet no one knew because symptoms are such unreliable indicators of health.

With less than 10% of nerves dedicated to feeling, there may be no warning signs for a heart attack either. No one knows what occluded blood vessels feel like – the first sign they are blocked is when a heart attack actually happens. And so with cancer; the day before diagnosis the person feels well, even though they are definitely not. It isn't an overnight event, but a long-term process, so timing is crucial in healthcare.

It takes most cancers 8–10 years to grow to 1 cm in size, but then they take off and require only 1.5 years more to grow to 3.5 cm. Mammography is one of the most specific cancer tests around, but as a stand-alone screening test it misses approximately 20% of all cancerous tumours. Early detection healthcare is not prevention.

Even when they become apparent, symptoms will not guarantee healing. Our magnificent bodies are designed mainly to *function*, not to always feel, and they will carry on as long as possible despite what we do to them.

You may have thought you were being preventative about your health by simply having regular "check-ups", but those tests are still looking for pathology in the early stages – disease that is already there. Prevention is very different to early detection of disease; preventative measures look for dis-function or disease long before it gets to the disease stage. By all means do not miss out on mammograms, pap smear tests or skin checks for melanoma; they are imperative for picking up cell changes that can indicate cancer at an early stage. But prevention is so much better than cure.

Below is a powerful exercise to get you thinking. If some test available to you revealed the *likelihood* of illness in your future, what changes would you make to improve your health and wellness?

Tick the Things You Would Do

☐ Eat better

☐ Relax more

☐ Exercise more

☐ Have chiropractic care

☐ Meditate

☐ Have massages

☐ See a naturopath

☐ See a nutritionist

☐ Take your health practitioner's advice more seriously

☐ Stop smoking

☐ Drink less alcohol

☐ Reduce or avoid taking painkillers or unnecessary medications/drugs

☐ Use your legs more than the car

☐ Stretch or do yoga

☐ See a counsellor or a psychologist

☐ Read more

☐ Work with or clean your environment or yourself with less chemicals

- ☐ Avoid artificial additives and preservatives in foods

- ☐ Spend more time with loved ones

- ☐ Laugh and listen to music

- ☐ Do a heavy-metal detox

- ☐ Create Feng Shui

- ☐ Remove mold

- ☐ Remove mercury fillings

- ☐ Meditate and do breath work

- ☐ Participate in biophilia

- ☐ Dance, sing, play, walk in nature, watch the sun rise and the moon set

- ☐ Forgive more and make peace

- ☐ Make love more

- ☐ Breathe deeper and slower

- ☐ Create better work-life balance

If you ticked *any* of these things why on earth aren't you already doing them *now*? Why wait for fear to motivate you to do what you *know* would improve the quality of your life?

These actions are not designed to treat cancer or illness, but they will certainly improve your health with or without disease and decrease your chances of ever contracting it. The secret is that if you are proactive about your health and wellness on a physical, chemical and social level, if you don't wait for symptoms in order to take action, then you will not become just another medical statistic, you will be a *vital* statistic. Prevention starts today. Let's go!

It's Easier to Stay Well than to Get Well

True health is not merely the absence of symptoms or disease. It's not just about living, but about having a tremendous *quality* of life. True health is in the adage "an ounce of prevention is worth a pound of cure". For centuries, we have based our health on appearances – if we *look* healthy, we must *be* healthy, right? Wrong! How many people have you known personally or read about in the media who appeared to be in the pink of health, and were later shocked to discover they had cancer? Even with the best laboratory procedures and a pill for every ill, even slender, young, athletic people can be unwell with no one the wiser.

It's a simple fact that prevention is better than cure – just ask anyone who is ill and in need of healing. The way of the future is a huge shift in consciousness from the "curing sickness" paradigm to the "maintaining wellness" paradigm, which is why alternative health therapies are becoming more main stream every day.

People are coming to realise that not only is it easier to stay well than to get well, it saves money and lives. Private healthcare funds now cover most alternative therapies as the demand grows for prevention rather than cure. Gone are the days when we "wait 'til it's broke to fix it". This is not because private insurers necessarily understand wellness. It is because there is a groundswell of consumers like you and us demanding preventative care.

Why the change? Well, it could have something to do with the fact that one in three people today will develop cancer at some time in their lives, and predictions that it will rise to *one in two* within the next decade. What is happening to the western world? As stress levels and medication use rise, our bodies are desperately trying to adapt both chemically and emotionally to the new environment we are creating.

The way we farm has also changed. In fact, we are not cooking and eating at home as often, let alone growing our own food and being sustainable. There has been a loss of connection for a long time now. Without prevention strategies, we are getting sicker, and increasingly fed up with medicines that simply mask symptoms without treating causes.

Medicine reigns supreme in emergency and sick care, but has little to offer in the field of *wellness*. When medicine fails us, we begin the search for the secrets to greater health.

If you want to really be well, rather than just not sick, then allopathy (orthodox medicine) is not for you.

Triumph over Illness

I recently asked a dentist what percentage of the population was familiar with the concept of bi-annual dental check-ups. He replied that around 90–100% of adults knew about it, but when we asked how many actually practiced it, he estimated 40%. Almost everyone knows it, yet only 4 out of 10 do it. Why? Because 6 out of 10 people judge their dental health on how they *feel*. But the day you have a raging toothache and get upset with the dental receptionist for not booking you in *immediately* is far too late. Since the last check-up your tooth had been slowly deteriorating, but because enamel has no nerve supply you felt ... nothing.

This is what happens when you *choose* to practise allopathy and only address your health when the symptoms appear. It's like putting off servicing your car until it breaks down on the side of the road, or not eating until you're starving. Of course, that's absurd, but most people approach their health that way, on a maintenance-basis only. You don't just brush your teeth when they hurt, you brush them every day. Let's apply that principle to every part of our body.

Allopathy doesn't respect the body's innate ability to heal itself when cared for properly, but of late there has been a movement toward "preventative" measures such as blood tests, full-body CT or MRI (Magnetic Resonance Imaging) scans, genetic tests and so on. This is not true wellness, because they are still looking for signs and symptoms of impending disease, just much earlier than they used to.

The concept is being so distorted that there are now women undergoing what are euphemistically called "prophylactic radical mastectomies". Yes, some women so fear even the possibility of developing breast cancer that they are having their perfectly healthy breasts cut off, *just in case*. Where will it end? Could future dentists decide that when a child's milk teeth fall out, it's more efficient to put in a complete set of dentures because the adult teeth will only develop cavities anyway?

When some women have a radical mastectomy, a surgeon may suggest that despite the lack of cancerous spread to any surrounding tissue, she should undergo preventative chemotherapy and radiotherapy as well as a five-year course of powerful toxic drugs, with all the life-afflicting side effects that it entails, "just in case" there were any cancer cells left. Many actually contemplate it — not because it is logical, but because of fear.

Your health choices should be contemplated and dictated by inspiration, evolution, and a desire for greater life, not the fear of disease or death.

You might feel this is prevention for you, but are you actually taking control of your own health too?

People who say they don't have time to take care of their health are absolutely right!

Dr Ben Lerner
Author of One Minute Wellness

This is Dr Lerner's humorous way of saying that if we don't care about or value something, we won't make time for it in our lives. It's not that we don't *have* time, we just don't *make* time.

Dr John F. Demartini, the world-renowned speaker and author on physical and mental health, has explored the science of motivation and success for decades. All his research has led him to state categorically that human beings are value-driven, and that their values dictate their destiny. This means you will be successful in the things that matter most to you, and unsuccessful in the things that matter least. It's not that you can't be successful in anything you really apply yourself to, but we only have so much time and energy, and your *values* will determine what you choose to give that time and energy to. This is a profound principle, and it can be the key to transformation in any area of your life that you choose. But don't take our word for it, do the exercise below and find out for yourself.

Exercise

Make a list of the 7 most important things in your life, the things you most care about and think about and give time to, the things that would most negatively impact you if they were suddenly taken away, such as children, family/loved one, job/ career, finance, intelligence, social, religion/spirituality, etc. Write them down in order from the most important to the least important and then look at where you have the most success and fulfilment.

IWw guarantee that the top three will be your areas of greatest achievement, and the further down the list the less successful you will be. If this isn't so for you, then the list you've written is probably not your true values, but what you think or assume or hope them to be. Look again, because if you don't give something your time, energy, thought, care and focus, it is not a true value for you.

It's a simple fact of human existence that we conduct our lives according to our values. For a mother, her children are usually higher on her value system than anything else and she will live and even die for them. If she has to choose between caring for and protecting them, and anyone or anything else, they win. To a high-flying professional, it's their work, and they will do anything for it. To a dedicated student, it's their study. To a top athlete, it's their strength, speed and nutrition. To a new love or newlyweds, it's ... well, you get the picture.

But for any of these people, if their health was severely challenged, they would immediately drop everything else and focus all their attention on getting better, because without good health the ability to appreciate any of the other values is vastly reduced. Isn't it strange that we are so committed to all the other values in our lives, but most of us take the precious gift of life itself for granted?

This is why in health and in life equally, we will need to be dynamic with our approach. What worked for us last week or last year, may not work for us this week or this year. Life is constantly changing and being aware and connected to ourselves, helps us to make healthy decisions on a holistic level that suits the world around us and what's happening for us in terms of our own personal evolution.

We live our lives according to our values. If wealth isn't in your top three, then don't expect to have much. If you don't put health high on your value list, don't expect to have it, or if you have it by simple virtue of youth, then don't expect to *keep* it.

It's the choices you make today that determine the quality of your life tomorrow.

Time is precious. Virtually everyone I have coached through knowledge and healthcare says that they want their life to be filled with pursuing their dreams, having a more purposeful life, meaningful relationships, better businesses that leave the planet better, exploring what the world has to offer, and being with loved ones. Caring for your health even when you already have it will not only improve the *quality* of your life, it will *prolong* it, so that you can have more of whatever you love.

So if you think you haven't the time to exercise, to see a preventative health practitioner, to chop up vegetables instead of microwaving a meal, just realise that the time you are "saving" might simply be subtracted from your life at its end, or even just the quality of your life. You're making choices every minute of every day, but you may not have been aware of exactly what you were choosing. Health just wasn't high enough on your value system ... until now.

The most unexpected thing that happens
to us is old age.
Count Leo Tolstoi

- To realise the value of ONE YEAR, ask a student who has failed a grade or a cancer patient with a year to live.

- To realise the value of ONE MONTH, ask a mother who has given birth to a premature baby.

- To realise the value of ONE WEEK, ask the editor of a weekly newspaper.

- To realise the value of ONE DAY, ask a daily wage labourer with children to feed.

- To realise the value of ONE HOUR, ask the lovers who are waiting to meet.

- To realise the value of ONE MINUTE, ask a person who has missed the train.

- To realise the value of ONE SECOND, ask a person who has avoided an accident.

- To realise the value of ONE MILLISECOND, ask the person who has just won a silver medal in the Olympics.

- To realise the value of ONE INSTANT, ask the chiropractor who just released the life trapped by a bone on a nerve.

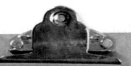

Time Suicide

by Dr Ben Lerner

Imagine you had a bank that credited your account each morning with $86,400, that carried over no balance from day to day, allowed you to keep no cash in your account, and every evening cancelled the amount you had failed to use during the day. What would you do? Draw out every cent, of course!

Well, you have such a bank, and its name is time. Every morning it credits you with 86,400 seconds. Every night it rules off as lost whatever you failed to invest to good purpose. It carries over no balances. It allows no overdrafts. Each day it opens a new account with you, and each night it burns the records of the previous day. If you fail to use the day's deposits, the loss is yours. There is no drawing against tomorrow. You must live in the present – on today's deposits. Invest it so as to get from it the utmost in health, happiness and success!

Life is not a possession, it's a *gift*, and if you don't value gifts you usually don't get more.

I once knew of a young man, a highly motivated entrepreneurial financial advisor, and during his consultation I found that his nervous and spine system were under immense stress and pressure. He went through the recommendations for his program of chiropractic care, and at the end he said, "Well, I guess that if I do this health thing, it would be like me saving money now in my 20s. But if I don't get adjusted and wait another 20 years, that's like beginning to save in my 40s. Financially, I know that's just not enough time, and it's much, much harder."

Connecting health and health care to your highest values (just like how he conducted his business) will motivate you to absorb and apply what you learn here. However, nothing of lasting value ever comes easily. At first, it can be quite disruptive (and therefore uncomfortable) to make changes in your lifestyle; you may have lived your whole life a certain way, and generations of your family before you, and old habits die hard.

But fortunately, no one expects you to do everything in this book all at once. It may take years to incorporate every concept into your new life, but each one changes you for the better. As you learn you'll grow wiser without having to grow old.

It's great to wake up to new knowledge, but there is no point in judging yourself for not listening to your body's warning signals sooner. We're only human – sometimes it takes a symptom or pain to get our attention and put us on a new path. And please understand that wellness is not about removing pain and symptoms. They are a vital part of the health process, so no matter what path you follow you won't ever reach a point where you will never have pain again.

If it wasn't for pain, we wouldn't be motivated to make changes. Read that again.

So decay can be painful, but so can growth – that's why they're called "growing pains". Just be aware of this as you begin to make changes in your life, and be grateful that any discomfort you experience comes from growth. The key to wellness is learning to listen to the warning signs, and being thankful that you can feel.

I once knew of an extraordinary man in chiropractic care whose entire spinal cord was riddled with cancer. His whole body was numb; he couldn't feel anything, and was completely unable to move. After just one chiropractic adjustment, he could wiggle his toes again, and feeling began to return, as his brain reconnected to the rest of his body. Prior to this, there was a blockage and distorted signals from his brain to the rest of his body.

All of a sudden, he expressed that he was still in pain, but he could now feel again. With tears in his eyes he said, "Thank you for this pain. The day you wake up not feeling anything is the day you are dead!" To him, feeling was everything. He was reconnected.

So far, we've talked about *what* prevention is and *why* it's so important. Now let's have a look at what it actually *is*, and what you can do to begin making a profound difference in your health.

Smoking: In the past there was some excuse to smoke; no one knew about the effects and the television was full of ads saying things like, "Seven out of ten doctors recommend filter cigarettes," and linking fine Virginia tobaccos with healthful relaxation, and even feminism! But we no longer have the excuse of ignorance.

Thousands of studies have revealed the effects of smoking on virtually every aspect of your health, from cancer of the mouth, lips, tongue, throat and lungs, to heart disease, emphysema, blood clots, gangrene, peripheral numbness, amputations, reduced oxygenation of the brain, reduced libido, premature ageing of the skin … the list is almost as extensive as the human anatomy itself.

It has been estimated that every cigarette takes 10 minutes off of your life, and the average smoker has a reduced lifespan of 10–12 years. If you choose to continue to smoke for the pleasure it gives you, then it's your choice. Just realise that you are shortening your lifespan and the multitude of pleasures you could have otherwise enjoyed.

Food: Ah, food! One of the greatest pleasures of life, and one of the greatest pains. The first change you may want to make is to *enjoy* it. With the growing consciousness about the benefits of healthy foods and the drawbacks of the alternatives, emotions have crept into the equation. Studies have been conducted on the consumption of "junk" foods, and to the astonishment of the researchers it was found that guilt about eating it had a more powerful depressant effect on people's immune systems than the food itself. So eat wisely, and well.

It's wise to cut down on take-away, pre-packaged and fried foods in order to reduce your intake of unnecessary fat and salt, and to increase the amount of fish (for the omega-3 oils), fresh fruit and vegetables in your diet. It's also wise to be conscious of not just the quality of what you eat, but also the quantity. Twenty years ago, statistics showed that the average person gained one pound per year after the age of 30 – today, it's *one kilogram*. That means by the age of 50, you will be, on average, 20 kilos heavier than you were at 30. Unless, of course, you do something about it now.

Slow down your eating, and savour every mouthful. There is an appetite "switch" in the hypothalamus of our brain that switches "on" when we're hungry, and "off" when we've had enough. However, there is a time delay before the fullness signal travels up the vagus nerve, via the blood supply, to the brain and tells it to turn off. Most of us eat so quickly that by the time the brain knows we're full and tells us to stop, we've eaten much more than we need. So slow down! Don't let the amount of food on your plate dictate your eating, stop when you've had enough. It's ironic that in the developed world, death from over-eating now exactly balances death from under-eating in the third world.

There is one more secret about food that I'd love to share with you. There have been many laboratory experiments on the effects of reduced nutrition, and the *most conservative* found that mice on a diet of 75% of their normal caloric intake lived 40% longer than their well-fed cage-mates. Eating, drinking and the process of digestion take a lot of energy, and release floods of free radicals (incomplete molecules) which race around the body damaging other cells and tissues. The ill effects of under-eating are as severe as those of over-eating, so do be moderate. As a general rule, if you eat *less*, you live *longer*. The types of calories are more important than the amount of calories too. You want to eat as close to nature as possible and organic where possible.

Stress: There is an old saying from the 60s, *"speed kills"*, and it applies not only to drugs but to driving and also lifestyle. The more stressed you allow yourself to become, the more you engage your sympathetic nervous system and adrenals, the higher your blood pressure, the more reactive your emotions, the shallower your breathing, and the less your appreciation of life. Stress also triggers the production of more cortisol, the so-called "stress chemical", which causes your body to crave carbohydrates, turns more of the food you eat into stored fat, and deposits more of that fat around your waist and organs.

If you have a stressful life, find ways to reduce or to cope with it; meditation, massage, music, walks in nature, weekends away, time with friends, walking the dog or petting the cat, holidays and quality down-time in solitude or with your loved ones, perhaps not pushing quite so hard or so long in the pursuit of your goals that you not only forget to smell the roses, you forget they even exist.

Regular medical, and chiropractic check-ups: Remember that an ounce of prevention really is worth a pound of cure. We have not yet adapted to walking fully upright, it's still a relatively new evolutionary step, and regular spinal adjustments can have the most extraordinary benefits for your wellbeing. Not only can you avoid major physical complications, you will increase your energy and vitality when all your systems are functioning optimally.

Hydration: You've been hearing about this for years, but do you know why you don't just do it? Some say they don't like the taste of water. Have you ever considered the quality of water you consume is not great? Or are you too busy and distracted that you forget? How can you make it convenient to remember? I have a Waters Co filtration and alkalising system in my home and it makes it really enticing and easy to hydrate. Drinking alkalised water helps neutralise acids and creates a structure and energy for cellular hydration to occur.

When you are out, you can fill up a steel flask or bottle. Avoid using plastics. They're really toxic. BPA-free bottles are fine. Drink plenty of pure, fresh water every day; 6–8 glasses is great. It will assist your digestion and elimination, help your cells to rid themselves of toxins, clear your eyes and skin, facilitate weight loss, and water is pH neutral (neither acid nor alkaline) which is the optimal state for radiant health.

The quality of water is everything too. Filtered and ionised water is incredible for wellness too. We are also dehydrated because we don't eat enough plants which also contain 70–80% water. Processed foods have no water content. Additionally, when we consume things like caffeine and alcohol, they're going to dehydrate. Cleansing and detoxing is a perfect way to boost detoxification systems, flush out toxins, hydrate cells, boost immunity and, of course, nourish your body. The human body can survive for a month without food but only a matter of days without water. It's a vital part of being well.

It helps to maintain a healthy body weight by increasing metabolism and regulating appetite. It also helps increase energy levels.

The most common cause of daytime fatigue is actually mild dehydration. A mere 2% drop in body water can trigger things like trouble with basic math, erratic behaviour, difficulty focusing, constipation and cravings for sugar, sweets and caffeine. Dehydration is a condition where the body's ability to operate as a self-healing organism is blocked. It affects blood pressure, blood sugar metabolism, digestion and kidney function. Headaches and fatigue are all signs of dehydration.

Studies show that 75% of Americans are chronically dehydrated and this statistic is likely applicable to the world's population. In 37% of Americans, the thirst mechanism is so weak, it is mistaken for hunger. It takes 4–6 weeks to rehydrate the body properly as it takes time to get out of dehydration mode which is equivalent to starvation made. The primary role of the body is survival so it will retreat into survival mode when it has been dehydrated for too long and begin to store water later.

Need more reasons to hydrate? What about the fact that most of us have access to it. Let's be grateful for something that is so nourishing.

Breathing: We all do it, but very few of us do it well. Most of us breathe shallowly, lifting our shoulders on the inhalation instead of extending our bellies (diaphragm), which results in "tight shoulder, loose abdomen" syndrome – exactly the opposite of what we want, which is "loose shoulder, firm abdomen". When we're hyper (excited), we tend to have long inhalations and short exhalations. When we're hypo (depressed), we tend to have long exhalations and short inhalations.

Optimal health and energy derive from a balanced one-to-one breath, where the inhalations are deep and regular and of exactly the same length. Spend just three minutes a day in a fresh-air environment, becoming aware of and re-educating your body's breathing rhythms and every part of you will benefit. If you try it and like it, consider taking the next step and enrolling in a yoga class to learn even more about *pranayam* (energy breathing), *nadis* (energy centres) and other esoterica. In the ancient Hindu tradition, the breath is a very old and extremely powerful technique to promote health of body and mind. Be connected to your breath.

So there you have just a few things you can do to dramatically improve your health and wellbeing. How can we be so sure? Well, apart from history, decades of medical studies, research and personal experience, even life insurance companies say so. They have compiled statistics on human behaviour for generations, they exist solely to make money and they dramatically reduce their premiums for non-smoking and healthy lifestyles. The longer you live, the more money they make, and they know that if you do these things, you will live longer.

These are the facts, and what you do with them is up to you. If you link these actions to your highest values, then your life will be transformed. Don't over-burden yourself, it's wiser to choose one thing at a time, become familiar and stable in it, and only then begin another. If you try to run before you walk, you'll only end up going back to the basics, so "make haste slowly".

The haste of a fool is the slowest thing in the world.
Thomas Shadwell

Everyone wants health, but some of us believe it is no longer possible for us. We sabotage ourselves with affirmations like, "It's too late for me", "It's just part of getting old", "Everybody has to put up with this", "My doctor says there's nothing he can do", "Who do you think you are?", "It's hereditary", and hundreds more. These thoughts have real power, they limit your potential and leave no room for change, making you a victim of limited personal, family and social beliefs.

We are committed to a revolution in human health, so that in the future no one needs to wait for disease (the tangled parachute) to tell them that something is amiss, and a vital step on that journey is a new understanding of health. If you've read this far, you are understanding the magnitude of the wellness concept and soon you will understand our wellness response, so here is an essential description of the tools that will help you on your way.

The "Health Journey"

- **Commitment.** Understanding that health is a quest, not a destination. It's a life-long process, not an event.

- **Knowledge.** Information and re-education as to what true health is.

- **Partnership.** Working with and listening to your carer, and ensuring that they want the same results you do, as some only seek symptom relief and not wellness care.

- **Patience.** Realising that there are limitations to matter. As our bodies replace cells daily and regenerate over time, healing is possible, but it may take longer than we think.

- **Trust.** Respecting that this process in motion (healing and health) will occur in the body's own timing, even though there are adjuncts that can fast track it.

Finally, some people believe that health and youthfulness are a matter of luck or good genetics, or that when they're gone, they're gone. None of this is true. An astonishing article was published in the scientific periodical, the *Journal of Vertebral Subluxation Research* (JVSR) on February 18th, 2005, and covered on the *Medical News Today* on March 7th of the same year. The breakthrough was the result of collaboration between chiropractors and researchers at the University of Lund, Sweden, and they discovered something amazing — chiropractic care influences basic physiological processes affecting oxidative stress and DNA repair.

What does this imply? Cell oxidation and DNA decay have long been known to be two of the key factors in ageing and physiological dysfunction, but chiropractic care has been clinically demonstrated to reverse and repair both. Genetics and past behaviour need no longer dictate our destiny, it's up to us, and we now have the most groundbreaking science to prove it. It may seem unbelievable, but it's true.

How to Get Connected

The only one responsible for your health is YOU so ...

- Don't blindly accept "authorities" as gospel, ask more and different questions.

- Do some research, find out for yourself.

- Get second or third opinions until you're satisfied.

- Don't be reactive to symptoms, "waiting 'til it's broke". Be proactive to health and listen to your body.

- Exercise more, stop smoking, eat well, drink more water, and breathe!

- Your health, your time, and your life are precious, treat them that way.

Share what you learn with your friends and loved ones, so you too can help them empower themselves with at least one secret and make them companions on your journey. After all, it's no fun keeping secrets like these to yourself.

Remember, you are responsible for the choices you make. Your doctor isn't responsible for your wellbeing, you are. It is truly up to you, and that's why it's imperative to take the time to plan your life and health.

In the next chapter, you'll learn about the powerful ally you have working with you – your own body's innate intelligence, and its ability to heal itself.

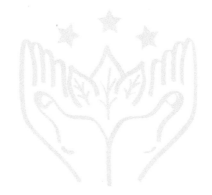

2

YOUR WELLNESS RESPONSE

Your Body
Self-Heals
and
Self-Regulates

*I am dying from the treatment
of too many physicians.*

Alexander the Great

This chapter is dedicated to exploring this question: who is the greatest healer, your doctor or your body?

The answer will be surprising, even amazing. It will help you to reclaim your power back and start to take full control of your health. Your health is in your hands.

In a very real sense, health is life itself – if you don't think so, just ask someone who has lost theirs. We go to doctors because we have an inherent desire for more and better-quality health and life, and we have been taught that only they can provide it for us. We don't even question that belief, but is it always true?

In fact, a doctor is an excellent assistant in your quest to fulfil your body's potential, but even he or she is on an ongoing quest to understanding how it actually works. Physicians may know a lot more than you about *what* it does, but how it does it is just as much a mystery to them as it is to you.

Think about this for a moment. Every single cell in your body undergoes six *trillion* chemical reactions per second, every second of your entire life, and they're all finely controlled. When you realise that your body consists of 100 trillion cells and 220 cell types, all working together in perfect harmony for seventy, eighty, even one hundred *years*, you begin to get an idea of how amazing your body really is.

The truth is that all of the most brilliant minds in the history of humanity, all working together, could not run a single human cell – it's just too complex. The greatest genius ever born does not have the mental capacity to manage a single cell, yet your body runs 100 trillion of them for up to 100 years.

On a very simple level, you know that a paper cut on your finger even without a band-aid or medication, will actually heal all by itself. It happens spontaneously, but does anyone actually know how to accomplish this extraordinary and complex feat of healing?

Of course not, but the body does. Healing happens inside us all the time on much more profound levels, but most of us are completely unaware of the physical magic our incredible bodies are performing all day, every day of our lives.

The Wellness Response is a healing and immune response and your body expressing wellness. Understanding symptoms as a vital part of the cure is what helps you change your perception on how to work with the body instead of fighting against it.

Self-Healing Power #1

Fever

When you get a cold, or a virus such as measles or chicken pox, there is often an accompanying fever, but did you ever stop to wonder why? Did you even realise that these illnesses are viruses?

One of the immune system's most effective weapons against illness is temperature. The viral cell wall is a very strong defensive barrier which is highly resistant to your immune system, so the body has developed a brilliant strategy to overcome this sneaky invader. Your normal body temperature is an ideal environment for illness, so raising your temperature with a fever is a beautifully orchestrated mechanism by which the body breaks down the wall and gains access to the virus itself, making it easy for the white blood cells to destroy it.

We are exposed to and have trillions of viruses every day. Are they friends and not so much foe?

It is an accepted belief that a fever is "bad" rather than part of a natural healing process, so modern medicine strives to reduce fevers, in direct opposition to the body's natural intelligence.

A change in core temperature is neither degenerative nor a sickness, it's an intelligent adaptation to a threat, and reducing fever with medication in this instance is working against that innate intelligence.

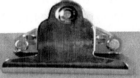

True Story

One day, a distraught mother burst into a chiropractic practice I once knew about, with the limp and feverish body of her 11-month-old daughter in her arms, begging to help the child.

As a trained nurse the mother considered herself a capable diagnostician, so on the Monday when her daughter developed a temperature of 38.5°, she gave her paracetamol to reduce the fever, which it did. Twelve hours later the fever rose again to 39°, so she took the little girl to her doctor who suggested another course of paracetamol, which over the next 12 hours reduced the fever again. This process was repeated for the next two days, with each episode typified by a dramatic increase in temperature, until she arrived on the chiropractor's doorstep with a temperature of 40.1°. This is a life-threatening and potentially fatal condition.

Her body's innate healing power had been trying to raise her body temperature to the point where the virus could be conquered, but each dose of paracetamol had interfered with and dangerously prolonged the body's innate healing process.

Let's explore this further.

Hippocrates was a Greek physician of the 4th century BC, now known as "the father of medicine". His discoveries are the basis of western medical understanding, and graduating doctors still take a version of the Hippocratic Oath today. Interestingly, the first principle they swear by is "to do no harm".

Surgeons and medical doctors have certainly done great good and saved millions of lives, but have they always strictly fulfilled this oath? It's not always their fault because this is just the way allopathic professionals are trained, but now we need to all work together and heal the divide between health modalities. A lot of the time there has been professional jealousy that I have witnessed and it has gotten in the way of true healing for the person. Let's remember the one who requires healing is the most important person in the relationship.

Let's look at the three leading causes of death in the western world. *Do you even know* what they are?

I often tell my clients, readers and audience the top three causes of death. Most people confidently give "heart disease and cancer" as the top two, then guess the third. When it is revealed that in fact heart attacks/disease and cancer come second and third in the death lottery, there is a moment of stunned silence, and then a forest of hands go up to ask what the number one cause of death could possibly be. No one has yet guessed the mystery health hazard that is more lethal than the big two. We are not talking bout Covid19 here.

Do *you* know the answer? If not, then why on earth not? After all, it's the leading cause of death in our world. The fact that people are completely oblivious to this hidden killer is one of the reasons I felt *compelled* to write this book, because you deserve to know.

So, what is the leading cause of death in our society? Would you be shocked to learn that the answer is ... *medical and hospital error*?

Well, it is, and there is even a term to describe this deadly phenomenon – *iatrogenesis*. Have you ever heard the word? Do you know what it means or even how to pronounce it? How is this possible? Why isn't it a daily topic of discussion? If it's the most likely single cause of your own death, it's certainly important enough.

Iatros is ancient Greek for "healer", and *genesis* means – "coming into being", so together the word literally means "made to happen or created by the healer". Iatrogenic illnesses are those created by a doctor, and the truth is that which we thought was the greatest source of health and healing is also the greatest cause of death. The facts speak for themselves.

The US reflects or anticipates the health statistics for the developed world, and in as early as 2001 official US government statistics reported the top three annual death rates as follows:

- **Cancer** – 553,251 people.

- **Heart disease** – 699,697 people.

- **Iatrogenesis** – 783,936 people dead.

It is self-evident that the American medical system is the *leading cause of death* and injury in the US. How is this possible?

Some forms of iatrogenesis are:

- misdiagnosis
- negligence or faulty procedures
- hospital or surgical error
- mis-prescription of medication
- pharmacist error
- radical treatments
- overuse of drugs leading to antibiotic resistance.

In all fairness, doctors themselves are not to blame for iatrogenesis. Our entire modern healthcare system and philosophy, however, *are* responsible for permitting and even promoting so many unnecessary procedures, drugs and mishaps. We also need to start taking responsibility for our own health and be more proactive when it comes to our own wellbeing. We cannot simply live an unhealthy lifestyle and wait for the best doctors and drugs to save us.

The Mayo Clinic, widely recognized as one of the most prestigious medical institutions in the world published how often misdiagnosis occurs.

Many patients come to Mayo Clinic for a second opinion or diagnosis confirmation before treatment for a complex condition. In a new study, Mayo Clinic reports that as many as 88 percent of those patients go home with a new or refined diagnosis -- changing their care plan and potentially their lives. Conversely, only 12 percent receive confirmation that the original diagnosis was complete and correct.

In 2015, the National Academy of Medicine reported that most people will receive an incorrect or late diagnosis at least once in their lives, sometimes with serious consequences. It cited one estimate that 12 million people — about 5 percent of adults who seek outpatient care — are misdiagnosed annually. The report also noted that diagnostic error is a relatively under-measured and understudied aspect of patient safety.

In 62 cases (21 percent), the second diagnosis was "distinctly different" from the first, the researchers reported. In 36 cases (12 percent), the diagnoses were the same. In the remaining 188 cases, the diagnoses were at least partly correct but were "better defined/refined" by the second opinion, according to the study.

Naessens and Graber said a second opinion is valuable any time a patient is told he or she has a serious condition, such as cancer, or needs surgery — even if an extra visit initially means more expense. In the long run, additional advice can save lives and money, they said.

"Doctors are humans, and they make the same cognitive mistakes we all make," Graber said.

Given the lack of public education about the abundance of preventive options now available, how are we to question the authorities in whose hands we place our lives and those of our loved ones? This illustrates precisely why our whole *system* is so desperately in need of change. A definitive study and close reading of medical peer-reviewed journals and government health statistics illustrates how American medicine frequently causes more harm than good.

- The number of people having in-hospital, adverse drug reactions (ADR) to prescribed medicine is 2.2 million. Dr Richard Besser, of the CDC, said in 1995 that the number of unnecessary antibiotics prescribed annually for viral infections was 20 million. Dr. Besser, in 2003, now refers to tens of millions of unnecessary antibiotics.

- The number of unnecessary medical and surgical procedures performed annually is 7.5 million.

- The number of people exposed to unnecessary hospitalisation annually is 8.9 million.

The American Medical Association admits that fully one half of all the money spent at the doors of healthcare providers – over 700 billion dollars last year – was for preventable problems.

Steven Shochat, DC

I wanted to discover specifics on iatrogenesis in Australia, but it seems there isn't enough information. I was introduced to someone who has spent quite some years on researching the topics and here is what Dr Michael McKibbon shared:

"Iatrogenesis in Australia is alive and well, pardon the pun! About twenty years ago, I was prompted to find out the mechanism preventing Australia's federal government from accurately reporting how many people die due to medical treatment as distinct from their disorder.

My journey of discovery included co-authoring a submission to the WA government, expressing concern that public patients are endangered by no accurate accounting of Australia's true total iatrogenic death toll. During the last twenty years, that and numerous supporting information has been circulated to Australia's mainstream media.

Politicians and the media meet that information with a uniform wall of silence.

Gary Null et al met with a similar response in the USA" see http://whale.to/a/null9.html

Michael McKibbin DC

This information certainly evokes strong emotional reactions in people reading it for the first time, and I was equally shocked when I encountered these statistics. If medical and hospital error is the leading cause of death in the modern world, are we to shun and turn our backs on the entire profession?

The answer is No. For the treatment of trauma and surgery such as organ replacement, modern medicine is unrivalled in its practice and procedures. However, we must question the belief that drugs, medication and surgery should be our first and primary source of healing. Your doctor does have an important role to play in your healthcare, but that role needs to change dramatically from what it is and has been for too long now. If you simply leave something too long and there are limitations of matter when it comes to healing, you just may not be able to always have success. We are only human. Errors happen. Although miracles can happen too. Your body is incredible.

The more you know about the workings of your incredibly effective and intelligent self-healing system, the more you will trust it. Most of us are woefully unaware or unappreciative of our body's capabilities, so let's look at some more examples.

Self-Healing Power #2

Expelling

When you pick up a germ, your body immediately mobilises to get rid of it, and the quickest way to expel germs is through an orifice – which is a hole like the mouth, nose, ears, bottom or even the pores of the skin. So when you get a cold, the quickest way to expel the germs is through sneezing or coughing. Therefore, coughing and sneezing are not part of the disease, they are actually a vital part of the cure.

If you don't understand this and try to "cure" yourself by taking medications that repress this process, then you may actually extend the time it takes to expel the germ, and prolong your illness. So working against the body's natural healing powers can not only make it sicker for longer, but sometimes it will simply find another way of getting rid of the germ. This may be through the pores of the skin, so instead of a simple cold or flu you may end up with rashes and even eczema. It needs to come out of somewhere!

Self-Healing Power #3

Mucus

Not only does mucus carry and remove the dead germs that have been killed by your immune system, your body also surrounds the living invaders with mucus so that you can expel them by coughing or sneezing.

Increased mucus production also protects the delicate lining of the lung and oesophageal tract from infection. Suppressing this response with anti-histamine medications can allow the infection to remain inside, becoming larger and more aggressive, and prevent your own immune system from healing you.

What might happen if we left those sneaky invaders in there for too long? Would it manifest into something more sinister eventually? Does having a cold help us to become more immune to other illnesses later, if we work with the body instead of against it? When you take the time to heal, you rest, drink more fluids, eat less and literally detox and purge. Think of this time as a reset, instead of always "soldiering on".

Self-Healing Power #4

Vomiting

It sometimes happens that two people go out for dinner, order the same meal, and are served the same tainted or toxic food. One of them is then up all night being violently ill, while the other displays no symptoms. Who is the healthier person? Strangely enough, it's the one whose body was sensitive enough to recognise the poison and purge it through vomiting. Rather than allow it to putrefy in the stomach to be processed and passed on to the kidneys, liver, brain and other tissues, the intelligence of your self-healing and self-regulating body chooses to simply get rid of it entirely.

Vomiting may not be pleasant in the short-term, and must always be monitored by a health professional, but if the alternative is long-term poisoning, then it is definitely the lesser of two evils.

The same thing happens with alcohol toxicity as a result of over-indulgence. You may believe you're just having a good time, but your brilliant body protects you from liver damage, brain cell destruction, and reduces the hangover by simply expelling what it knows is poisoning you. We will learn more about alcohol toxicity in the following chapters.

It's important to respect the intelligence of your body and not work against your natural healing processes unless you are in a life-threatening situation, and that is something your primary healthcare practitioner can educate you about.

A modern mystery is the recent phenomenal rise of allergies and auto-immune diseases, and there are almost as many theories as there are social commentators. The connection between poor hygiene and disease has been known for centuries, but taking it too far may carry its own risks.

The medical profession, while responsibly educating the public about the importance of cleanliness, has also played an unwitting role in the unprecedented levels of antiseptic and even germ-phobic conditions in the average household. The "Hygiene Hypothesis" says that this has had a catastrophic effect.

Rapidly gaining credence, this theory says that the lack of normal challenge to our children's immune systems has sent them into overdrive, causing them to either overreact with allergic symptoms to normally benign substances in the environment or diet such as nuts, bread, dairy products and even *dust*, or to actually turn on the children themselves with life-threatening auto-immune responses.

Why do so many children, at a very early stage of their growth, sit and eat dirt whenever they get the chance? Don't you find this fascinating to watch? In countries all over the world, children eat dirt because they are genetically programmed to pick up both germs and antibodies, and develop resistance that way. The body *knows*, but we think we know better, and pay the price for our lack of trust and understanding. We will also uncover in the following chapters, what else babies need to thrive and discover how we come into the world is a vital part of our health.

Self-Healing Power #5

Rashes

Your skin is the largest organ in your body, and it performs many functions. It cools the body by sweating, contains innumerable sensory nerves that allow you to feel both pain and pleasure in order to negotiate your environment, carries beneficial bacteria, as a permeable membrane it lets beneficial matter in and waste products out, and so on.

Another vital role is to protect the sensitive internal body from the external pollutant world, which is why we take care not to allow cuts or wounds to become infected.

Your skin is a *carrier* as well as a barrier. The pores can absorb creams, liquids, dirt, pollution, basically everything that touches your skin.

Some personal hygiene products like make-up and moisturisers contain harmful chemicals which may be absorbed and accumulate in the body, causing long-term damage.

Parabens and sodium laurel sulphate (SLS – the ingredient that causes products to foam, such as soap, toothpaste, shampoos, shaving cream) have been known to cause skin reactions, and many companies now advertise their products as "paraben and SLS free".

It is best to avoid these paraben and SLS products even if you have no overt reactions, and if you do, realise that the reactions are actually healthy responses protecting you from much more serious organ and tissue damage.

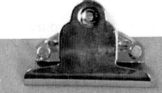

True Story

A little boy I once knew was receiving care at a wellness centre I worked in, and he developed a severe and extremely painful case of eczema. On consultation with his mother, it was found that she used a range of products containing parabens and sodium laurel sulphate. When she bathed him in warm water it nicely opened up all his pores, and his skin then simply drank up all the carcinogenic chemicals contained in the soaps and creams. His healthy little body simply didn't like it, and the eczematous rash that developed was a result of his body's intelligent self-healing mechanism that pushed the chemicals back out through the pores, rather than allow them to reach his organs and do even greater damage.

Prescribing a cortisone cream to force the chemicals back in would have disrespected his body's intelligence, and the reason it developed the rash in the first place. What was done instead was to simply make sure his mother used only paraben- and SLS-free soaps and creams, and the condition soon completely cleared up without any chemical intervention.

This addressed the cause rather than merely fixing the symptom. He was suffering from an excess of chemicals, and he certainly didn't need to be cured with more.

For decades, alternative health practitioners, as well as a farsighted minority in the medical profession, have been speaking out against the widespread overuse of antibiotics.

Developed in the 1930s, these "wonder drugs" have saved millions of lives and quite rightly are consistently listed among the greatest discoveries of all time.

However, while deadly to most bacteria, antibiotics are completely ineffective against all viruses, such as colds and flus, which has not stopped their prescription in vast quantities for those very ailments, a deadly side effect of which has been the widespread exposure of countless micro-organisms to sub-lethal doses of antibiotics, allowing them to develop resistance to our most powerful medical weapon.

Conventional antibiotics are now quite ineffective against these "super bugs" and scientists are forced to develop ever new and more powerful variants to deal with them, hoping they can keep ahead of the problem. Golden staph is a well-known example of this phenomenon – highly resistant, difficult to cure, and hospitals throughout the developed world have themselves become breeding grounds for the infection.

Current statistics also reveal another clear and shocking fact – the greater the number of doctors in a community, the higher the death rate. As a result of studies conducted over decades, it's a well-documented (but not well-publicised) fact that mortality rates in a community are in direct proportion to the number of doctors there. The *more* doctors, the *higher* the death rate. And in communities with a historically low mortality rate, the death statistics *rose* as the numbers of doctors increased over time. This is an absolute contradiction to the unquestioned belief that outside resources should be our first and last resort for health, wellbeing and life itself.

It's not exactly a secret, but neither is it common knowledge. Somehow, you weren't told that going to the hospital is statistically more likely to kill you than cancer or heart disease. If you really think about iatrogenesis, you'll see why I take our role as a health and wellness educator so seriously. If you know that the treatment for a life-threatening disease may harm or even kill you, then you'll realise that it's safer, smarter and easier to stay well than to try to get well.

But what happens when, like most people, we ignore our body's miraculous self-healing and self-regulating capacity for too long?

We get sick. The body is so incredible at adapting, but there are limitations of matter and it can only adapt for so long. When we get sick, we blame some cause outside us, and we look for someone or something outside us to make us well again. We haven't cared or known enough to *stay well*, so we suddenly need to *get well*. "Getting well" for many means simply returning to a state free from symptoms or disease, without addressing why they became sick in the first place or what they can do to prevent its recurrence. Is this true health though?

Often it takes a life-threatening illness to make us finally choose to change our lifestyle, which was actually the original "cause" of the illness. Wellness is about not only recovering, but also making lifestyle changes to go that one step further to prevent any possible relapse.

If you wait for too long, if you do nothing until illness manifests, then by default you are *choosing* to rely on medical intervention to "save" you. It's then up to you to make the necessary changes, which means taking responsibility for co-managing your life with all of your chosen healthcare providers to be the healthiest person you can possibly be.

Symptoms are not *bad*; they are a message from the body to the mind telling us that something requires our attention. The mind and body are not two, they are one, and when we ignore that truth there are always consequences.

I would rather know what kind of person has a disease, than what kind of disease a person has.

Hippocrates

Much of this information is a revelation to most people – they simply didn't know any better. Well, now you're beginning to, so what will you do about it? Prevention should be rising on your list of values, as reliance on medical intervention and "miracle" cures is dropping. There are so many situations where a properly cared-for body can heal itself, and it's up to you to learn more about your amazing organism so you can express better health.

Self-Healing Power #6

Cancer

So far, we've been questioning beliefs and gently pushing envelopes in our quest to inform and inspire you to take more responsibility for your own health and wellbeing, and now we're going to take a quantum leap.

Please keep in mind that this is an extraordinary story about a unique situation, and by no means is this book suggesting or recommending that anyone should turn their back on the skills and knowledge of the medical profession. If not for them we would have a much lower quality of life, and many people alive today would not be. I only include it as a story and example to illustrate the self-healing power of the human body, and to give you an idea of what has been and may be possible.

Scientist, speaker, teacher and contributor on *The Secret* who also conducts a seminar called "The Breakthrough Experience", Dr John F. Demartini, helps people resolve emotional charges and reclaim their personal power. Some years ago, a man came to that program with cancer of the throat. The tumour was on the left side of his neck, and he was about to undergo surgery to have his larynx and much of his throat removed.

Dr Demartini knew that the left side of the body relates to the feminine, while the right is masculine, and that a contributing factor in cancer can be long-term resentment or anger.

He asked the man what female was or had been controlling his life, and the man replied, "Well, take your pick. My mother dominated me, then my wife took over when I got married, we have four teenage daughters, and my mother-in-law lives with us. My whole *life* is run by women!"

The man's strongest resentment was towards his mother, so that weekend he opened up his heart to love her again, and thanked her for her contribution to his life. He underwent such a deep emotional catharsis that Dr Demartini suggested if it were possible, he postpone his surgery for a month to focus on resolving his issues with all the women in his life. When the man told his doctor of his decision he was told, "This is a very advanced and dangerous tumour. I strongly urge you to have the surgery immediately, and won't be responsible for the consequences of any delay."

But he delayed anyway and spent a month working on his relationship issues, and when he returned to his doctor, he was flabbergasted. There was absolutely no trace of the tumour. The doctor took a biopsy from the former site of the cancer and called him back in when the tests were done. He said, "I don't know what's going on here, but you are utterly cancer free. According to medical science, this is impossible. I can't explain it, I can only suppose that we must have misdiagnosed your condition originally." He shook his head, and sent him on his way with instructions to return in a few months for a follow-up examination.

That cancer never did return. The healing power of love and the wisdom of the body combined to cure him so profoundly and quickly that science called it "impossible" and discounted the entire phenomenon because it simply could not explain such a "miraculous" cure.

Take this story as a testament to the power that made the body and heals the body. Often there have been cases of this in people curing all sorts of illness with mindset and lifestyle changes. We will explore how perception, love and forgiveness can also play a part in our health.

I also had a similar experience a few years ago when I had an overdue pap smear test with my medical doctor. She detected low grade cancer cells in my cervix. There were abnormal cells and a lesion sighted. My medical doctor knew that I am interested in natural healing. She gave me six months to heal, and said that when we did another test, if there were no changes, we would have to start treatment. Within this six months, I looked at every angle of my wellness. My diet and lifestyle was clean. Where I needed to heal further was some trauma I needed to finally heal for that area to be well again. I discovered new modalities including kinesiology and worked on self-love and forgiveness. Six months later, of course I was a wreck. The nerves took over as I waited for my results, but it came back all clear. Even I couldn't believe the miracles that sometimes occur when we give our bodies the right energy and environment to heal.

This is why we must work together to support each other in what we believe is right for us. There are so many paths to wellness and loving each other harder is going to not only assist healing but also heal the divide amongst us all. Let's respect how individually unique we all are.

Remember, symptoms, disease and illness are not bad, they are *messages* from the body trying to reveal to us that something is not in order. If we really want to embrace our body's true capacity for healing, it's time to release the old and deeply entrenched misunderstanding of symptoms as enemies to be fought and overcome. As with the fever we discussed earlier, symptoms are the responses of our body's innate intelligence helping us to adapt to the challenge or stress we are facing. If we don't understand the message, we'll try and remove the symptoms. But if we learn how to listen to and decode the messages, then we can achieve an even greater degree of mental and physical health. This is why social, emotional and spiritual health (whatever higher force you believe runs us) is important to nurture too.

Self-Healing Power #7

The Heart

I've saved the best for last. Love is everything. I have played cupid and even been on shows and written a book about healthy relationships. The health of the heart is paramount. We know that heart disease is the second biggest killer in our society, and this is a story of the power of the human heart to heal itself.

Back in the 70s, in the early days of heart surgery, Dr Denton Cooley was performing open-heart surgery and heart transplants in Texas, and was widely regarded as a world-leader in his field. For some reason, his operations were unusually successful – his patients had fewer complications, less infections, a lower incidence of rejection, and a significantly higher survival rate. It was thought that it was due to his equipment, or perhaps his techniques, so many doctors from around the world came to study with him. What they found was amazing because the great difference was not what he *did*, but what he *said*.

When each patient had regained consciousness after surgery, he made it a point to visit them in their room. He would sit down on the edge of the bed, take their hand in his and look into their eyes, and say with absolute conviction and sincerity, "Mr. Jones, I just want to let you know that your surgery was a magnificent success. I'm proud of you. Soon you'll be able to hold your granddaughter in your arms again, and get back into your garden because I know how much you love to grow roses. I want you to know that soon you'll be hugging your wife again and telling her how much you love her. You're going to be fine now. I love having patients like you. Thank you."

He would not stop until they got tears in their eyes, their hearts opened, and they cried. Those were tears not of sadness but of gratitude – to him, and for life itself. Please also keep in mind that tears have analgesic properties. Crying can be completely healing if it's a release. Can you imagine the generations of people and indeed men who have been told it is not okay to cry?

That was his secret – not the technology, but the *humanity*. He was an example of a great doctor who understood the power of the human heart, not just the organ but the consciousness, and that made him a *healer*. He took the time to know his patients, to find out what moved and inspired them, what they really cared about and what connected them to life, and he used it to help them heal themselves. If you want to heal yourself, you would be wise to follow his example.

> *Doctors are the servant of the patient,*
> *not the master.*
>
> **Hippocrates**

The body is very resilient and forgiving, so by the time disease manifests you must have not only ignored your body's messages, but your doctor's repeated warnings as well. "Exercise is a great deterrent to heart disease. That unhealthy diet makes diabetes a real danger for you. Stop smoking." If you don't feel responsible for your own health and wellbeing, warnings like these are just water off a duck's back.

Obesity and smoking are the number one and number two causes of preventable death, and prime factors in many illnesses as well. If we're used to waiting until something is broken to fix it and then rely on an "expert" to do the repairs, then the facts about iatrogenesis show us that it may just be too late. Too many of us don't listen to our magnificent bodies, and instead we listen to some professionals who lead us to believe we are powerless without their help.

So, are you thinking of turning your back on doctors and surgeons, living on raw vegetables and cold baths, and relying solely on your own mind and body to keep you healthy?

Absolutely do not!

The wise person uses every possible means to maintain their health, just as a skilled painter doesn't rely on only a few colours, but uses the entire palette to create a masterful work of art. So too should you make wise use of the entire spectrum of medical experts and practitioners available to help you maximise your health. That means working in conjunction with them, selecting the ones that best suit you, and paying attention to the symptomatic warning lights that come on from time to time and seeking appropriate care.

The word "doctor" actually means "teacher" – the best doctors are not only skilled healers, they are also teachers. So choose yours wisely, listen to the advice they give you, and ask more questions to move from a passive "patient" to an informed co-manager of your own health.

What I definitely am *not* recommending is what most people do – to unconsciously rely on the body's resilience and powers until it breaks down, and then run to a doctor and ask them to clean up the mess. That is unwise, and unfair to both the doctor and your body.

If you don't give your body the nutrition, rest, care, and mental attitude it requires, don't expect it to give you its best. We've seen that prevention is better than cure, and that it's easier to stay well than get well. However, we sometimes hear wild claims made by the more extreme advocates that it is possible to wish our way to a perfect, permanent wellness. There is absolutely no evidence to support this belief. Sickness and death are part of life; they're not bad or wrong, they are there to put us back on track and value every day that we are blessed to be alive. But while you're here you can definitely optimise your life.

In ancient China, healers knew this; they saw themselves as servants and facilitators of the life force within us all. They called it *ch'i*, and took their responsibility so seriously that if you became ill, they would pay *you* because they hadn't done their job of maximising your body's self-healing capacity.

The best way to heal is to respect and maximise the body's self-healing and self-regulating functions. There are now excellent doctors available who can help you do this – they are integrative; they combine natural therapies into their care plan, and they help you get better without resorting to medication as their first port of call. They do this by thorough testing, and by working hand in hand with you (because *you* are the world's leading authority on you) and other professionals such as naturopaths and wellness chiropractors to make sure you get well and stay well.

Each and every day throughout your entire life, your body is performing miracles of self-regulation and healing. Without you giving it a second thought, cuts and wounds heal, hangovers fade, food is turned into energy, each cell is fed with oxygen and cleansed of carbon dioxide, your lymphatic system removes all the toxic by-products of cell activity, viruses and bacteria are overcome and expelled, illnesses and diseases are cured, overall homeostasis (balance of all systems) is maintained, cell breakdown and the ageing process are managed, symptoms are continually communicating with you (and mostly ignored or misunderstood), in women the miracle of gestation and birth is somehow accomplished, an incredible 300 million cells die and are replaced every *minute*, everything acts and interacts with inconceivable complexity, and it all goes on for *decades*, no matter how carelessly you treat your miraculous vehicle. There is a *vast* intelligence running this body of yours, and it is wise to be grateful and humble to an intelligence greater than our own.

Through the process of developing and then conquering infection, the child gets rid of acquired toxins and poisons from the body and receives a boost to the immune system.

Robin Hayfield
The Family Homeopath Healing

Symptoms and Disease

As a result of all the side, delayed and cumulative effects we're experiencing these days, the paradigm in healthcare is gradually moving from a symptom-based model to one in which the function, performance and innate healing potential of the human body is maximised. With this change in approach comes the realisation that not only are many diseases normal and natural, they may actually benefit the body by strengthening the immune system.

Using medicines to interfere with the normal progression of a disease, or injecting vaccines to anticipate the natural immune process, may be based on a limited or potentially biased understanding of the body and its healing potential, as well as an underestimation of the side effects of these treatments.

. Whenever the immune system successfully deals with an infection, it emerges from the experience stronger and better able to confront similar threats in the future. Our immune system develops in combat. If at the first sign of infection, you always jump in with antibiotics, you do not give the immune system a chance to grow stronger.

Andrew T. Weil
Spontaneous Healing

In an effort to keep your nerve system clean and functioning at peak efficiency, you may want to limit the introduction of unnatural substances in your body.

There is now a strong and growing movement of families choosing not to have vaccinations and rather opting for these viable alternatives. I do not have an opinion on what is best, as I believe that each person is unique, and health and healing needs to be practiced with the informed consent of the person, as they will decide and have the right to choose what works best for them, based on all that knowledge they're presented with. If you are curious about natural immunisation, then you may like to look into this further.

Use what is shared with you here as inspiration and a springboard to find out more about this amazing vehicle that you have been given – your human body.

Up until 1895, medical men said all disease was caused by bad, impure, stagnated, or hindered blood flow.

B.J. Palmer, DC, PhC

Perception in part determines our reality, and our perception is based on not only what we were taught by our parents and environment, but also the constant flow of information we receive through our senses.

At its core, this book is all about questioning the conditioning we have been brought up to believe in, and using our innate intelligence to find our own truths. What is your truth? It will be different to everyone else's and that's okay. There is unity in diversity, remember?

Wisdom begins with two things – questions and an open mind, so here are three powerful questions for you:

- With all our technological advances, why are more people dying of cancer and new illnesses every year?

- If the allopathic (medical) model is so effective, why do more people remain at risk of death as a result of medical and hospital error (iatrogenesis) than cancer, heart disease, or car accidents?

- And finally, what do you really base your healthcare decisions on – blind faith or knowledge?

In the very final chapter, we're going to be looking at another vital component in your life, which I can't wait for you to read, that may play a part in illness and wellness – your mind. It is time to create a paradigm shift in how we all viewed health.

The most important message to gain from this chapter is the value of knowing and trusting your body, and the power of prevention rather than maintenance.

Prevention goes beyond simply maintaining health to *improving* it, and there is no ceiling as to how healthy we can be. You have the potential for a life of health beyond anything you've every dreamed of.

Healthy Changes You Can Make

- Find a doctor who is open to natural therapies so that they can work with you and try to change the notion of needing to prescribe medication as a first option, as well as to explore the cause of the health challenge you are experiencing.

- Assess which health professionals are most suitable for you, in practice and philosophy.

- If in doubt, make sure your doctor is knowledgeable in natural therapies and can point you in the right direction.

- Make sure your doctor has a network of natural therapists who you can be co-managed with.

- Take proactive and preventative steps to improve your health and wellness on an emotional, chemical, physical and social level.

- Don't shun the medical profession; make sure you can work together as a team. After all, it's your body that will be doing the real healing.

- Do some research. When you make a healthcare decision, make sure it's based on knowledge, not blind obedience.

- Question authorities. Apply what you learn in your research to get the most out of your healthcare practitioners.

- Examine the alternatives to toxins such as homeopathic immunisation and overall strengthening of your immune system.

- If you choose to vaccinate yourself or your child, visit a wellness chiropractor immediately afterward to ensure that your nervous system is working at its best and is able to deal with the chemical stressor that has been placed upon it.

The truth is you have inside you an amazing ability to be well, healthy and vital from the day you enter this world until the day you leave it, *without* drugs and surgery – provided you make the right health choices.

So how can you be healthier without having to put anything into your body, or take anything out? By relying upon the powerful and intelligent healer you were blessed with from the very beginning. It's been with you all along; during foetal development it is the first system to appear, in the seventh hour of your body's formation, and we're going to explore its powers in the next chapter. What is this secret healer? Your nervous system.

References

Articles

Incidence of adverse drug reactions in hospitalized patients.

Lazarou J, Pomeranz B, Corey P. JAMA. 1998; 279: 1200–1205

Caution About Overuse of Antibiotics.

Rabin R. Newsday. Sept. 18, 2003

Investigation. Cost and quality of Health Care. Unneccessary Surgery.

US Congressional House Subcommittee Oversight. Washington, DC: Government Printing Office, 1976

Inappropriate Use of Hospitals in a randomized trial of health insurance plans.

Sonnenberg FA, Manning WG, Goldberg GA. Bloomfield ES, Newhouse JP, Brook RH, NEJM. 1986 Nov 13; 315 (20): 1259–66 and (94)

Patient, provider and hospital characteristics associated with Inappropriate Hospitilization.

Sonnenberg FA, Manning WG, Benjamin B. Am J Public Health. 1990 Oct; 80 (10): 1253–6

The cost of inappropriate admissions: a study of health benefits and resource utilization in a department of internal medicine.

Erikson BO, Kristienson IS, Nord E, Pape JF, Almdahl SM, Hensrud A, Jaeger S. J Intern Med. 1999 Oct; 246 (4): 379–87

Will More Doctors Increase or Decrease Death Rates? An econometric analysis of Australian mortality statistics.

Jeff Richardson, Stuart Peacock, Centre for Health Program Evaluation, Monash University. Working Paper 137, April 2003

Economics and Health System Reform.

Jeff Richardson, Australian Health Care Summit, Canberra, 17–19 August 2003

https://www.washingtonpost.com/national/health-science/20-percent-of-patients-with-serious-conditions-are-first-misdiagnosed-study-says/2017/04/03/e386982a-189f-11e7-9887-1a5314b56a08_story.html

https://www.sciencedaily.com/releases/2017/04/170404084442.htm

Websites

Centers for Disease Control and Prevention
www.cdc.gov/drugresistance/community http//.hcup/ahrq.gov/HCUPnet.asp

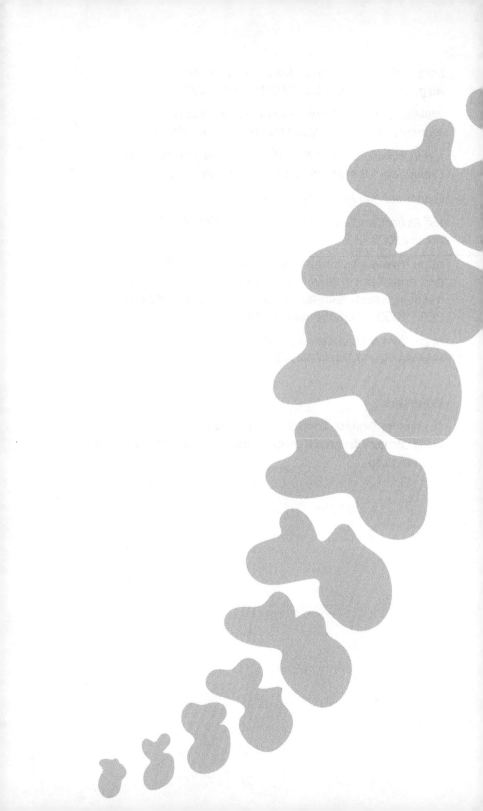

3

YOUR SPINE IS THE WINDOW TO YOUR HEALTH

*Chiropractic is so simple,
it's hard to believe.*

Ernie Landi, DC

Well, so far in just two chapters we've accomplished quite a lot. We've looked at the true nature of health and healing, some potential drawbacks of the modern medical system, the cost of waiting for disease to manifest before attempting to cure it, the importance of taking responsibility for your own health, the value of a preventive approach, and your body's incredible ability to heal itself.

Now let's take the next step and explore something that is near and dear to my heart, a revolutionary approach that has brought health not only to me and my clients personally, but to thousands of people, patients, and literally millions of people all over the world.

I can't believe some still do not know about this extraordinary healing modality which can dramatically improve the quality of your life and that of your family. Those fortunate enough to have experienced it never look back and continue with its care for life, while many who have not tried it are curious about what makes its supporters so enthusiastic in their praise. What is this "hidden health secret"?

I am talking about *chiropractic*, of course, and by the end of this chapter you will understand why I value it so highly and what a natural, gentle and yet extremely powerful force for healing it can be. I have been having chiropractic care for twenty years and have been getting checked weekly. No matter where I have travelled, I have made sure I have gotten off the plane and found a chiropractor to get checked before I went on to holiday or to work. I can say emphatically that it is the one thing that might be missing from your "healthy habits" that made the hugest difference tom my immunity, my age and my overall wellness.

We're going to be looking at why some have misunderstood this profession, how those perceptions are changing by leaps and bounds (quite literally),

Let's start with the basics — what *is* chiropractic, and where did it come from? The art of chiropractic is actually thousands of years old, and some of its techniques are described in the earliest writings of the Chinese. Over time, it was forgotten and became a long-lost art, and then re-emerged in the west over a century ago.

In 1895, Dr D.D. Palmer became dissatisfied with merely reacting to and treating his patients' symptoms. He wanted to find the cause of disease itself, and constantly explored many different healing disciplines.

One day, his janitor, who had been deaf for many years, allowed Palmer to examine him. The doctor noticed a lump in the man's neck, and inquired about how and when it first appeared. He then asked him when his deafness began, and learned that they were simultaneous events. Surprised that no one had ever made the connection before, and intrigued by the implications, he began to experiment. Examining the lump, Palmer believed he could feel a spinal bone out of alignment with the others, and convinced the janitor to let him attempt to adjust the shifted bone back into its normal position with his hands. To the astonishment of both men the bone moved, the janitor's hearing was restored, and chiropractic as we know it was born. It has grown rapidly, widely, and ever more deeply since that humble beginning, and is now a double science degree obtained at university level.

Chiropractic is the second largest primary healthcare profession in the United States, and the fastest-growing primary healthcare profession in the world that doesn't use drugs or surgery or anything that needs to be ingested!

**Chiropractic Science and Practice in the United States,
The International Chiropractors Association, 1991**

Being a primary healthcare practitioner means you don't need a referral to see them. It's your first stop, as they're trained in diagnostics too. In fact, chiropractors spend more hours in diagnostics than general practice medical doctors.

Strangely enough, the healing art and science of chiropractic is actually not a cure or treatment for anything. Put as simply as possible, chiropractic works by relieving interference to your nerve system, which allows your body to regain the natural healthy functioning it was designed to have. But if it's so beneficial, why are there so many myths and misconceptions about chiropractic? And don't forget that it is the medical model that has taught us to treat and cure, but chiropractic is rather about restoring function and allowing your body to do the healing, in whatever way that might be. We will learn more how that happens soon, but you can see where the misconceptions lie about claims that it cures anything.

To understand how such misunderstanding could come about, we also need to look at history. In the past, some healthcare practitioners didn't know exactly what chiropractors did, and mystery often creates mistrust. Upon hearing that ailments they themselves found so difficult to treat, such as asthma, colic and headaches, simply disappeared after chiropractic care, a natural professional jealousy grew. Sometimes, it was based in that mistaken belief that chiropractors were claiming to cure these diseases, when in fact they did not, they merely assisted the body to heal itself.

Early chiropractors themselves must also bear some responsibility for the confusion, because they achieved such extraordinary results with a multitude of diseases and ailments including common headaches, neck and back pain that they began to promote themselves for those treatments alone.

In addition, chiropractic became so successful that unqualified manipulative therapist practitioners jumped on the bandwagon and tried to emulate the techniques without understanding the exact scientific principles on which they are based, with varying results.

Fortunately, these growing pains have passed, and today's high standards require all practising chiropractors in Australia to attain the five-year double science degree and be registered with the Chiropractic Association of Australia.

The old rivalry is being superseded by a new spirit of cooperation as general practitioners find their patients asking them to work together with their chiropractor to experience the value and unique contribution to their clients' recovery.

Chiropractic has become a respected and integral part of the community by clarifying the chiropractic message to better serve the community and to fulfil its core purpose, which is to allow the body to heal itself at its true potential through proper functioning of the nerve system. They're an allied health professional, and an essential service as they keep people out of the hospital system.

The Spine

Chiropractic focuses on the nervous system and the spine as the centre of your being and healing with good reason. It is the most complex structure created by nature, and has given rise not only to human beings, but to all of their most powerful and subtle creations in turn.

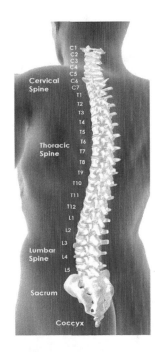

We humans spend months, years, even decades building structures such as buildings, dams and bridges which can withstand everything nature throws at them – cyclones, hurricanes, tidal waves, even earthquakes. The engineering is phenomenal, the architects are highly respected throughout the world, and often down through the ages, and all these creations are built around a structural spine.

Look at the Sydney Harbour Bridge, for example; it has an amazing structural spine, reinforced by over 6 million hand driven rivets, making it one of the most riveting sights in the world (apologies for the pun). It was designed to withstand the daily pressures of heavy traffic, weather, ocean movements and earthquakes, but it can't continue to do this, unchecked, throughout time.

A huge range of professionals and workers constantly maintain this architectural marvel; checking and monitoring, repairing, replacing, upgrading, painting, etc. If the stresses are not exactly aligned and integrated, down it comes. With so much pride in the bridge, preventative measures are taken daily to care for that vast spine, and yet ... most of us don't do the same for ourselves.

SPINAL LEVEL	BODY PAIN	INTERNAL ORGANS, FUNCTIONS & EFFECTS	COMMON INTERNAL SYMPTOMS INDICATING DIS-EASE
C1	Headache	Food Sensitivity, Structures of the Head	Spacey, dizzy, low energy, memory trouble, brain fog, sore throat, colds/flu, ear ache, etc.
C2		Sinuses	Sinus problems, snoring
C3	Neck	Diaphragm	Difficult to take a deep breath, chronic fatigue, anxiety, vertigo, shortness of breath
C4		Thyroid	Low = weight gain, feelings of being cold High = insomnia, nervous
C5	Shoulder	Sugar Handling	Craving sweets, tired after eating, headaches if too long between meals, emotional instability, heart palpitations
C6	Arm	Stomach	Stomach pain after eating, needs antacids
C7	Hand	Liver	Sluggishness, sneezing, nightmares, burning feet
T1/2	Finger	Heart	Coronary heart disease, functional heart conditions, chest pain
T3		Lungs & Bronchi	Bronchial asthma, shortness of breath, chronic cough
T4	Upper back	Gall Bladder	Heartburn, bloating after meals, gassy, burping, trouble with fatty foods
T5		Stomach	Heartburn, indigestion, stomach troubles, ulcers
T6		Pancreas	Craving sweets, indigestion, tired after eating, heart palpitations, emotional instability, headaches if too long between meals,
T7	Mid back	Spleen & Immune Function	Lowered resistance, immune deficiencies, frequent colds / flues
T8		Liver	Headaches, low energy, sneezing, nightmares, burning feet
T9		Adrenal Glands	Overwhelmed by stress
T10		Small Intestine	Digestive complaints: 1-2 hours after eating
T11/12		Kidneys & Bladder	Decreased urine output, swollen ankles, puffy eyelids, kidney or bladder infections
L1	Low back	Ileocecal Valve	Bad breath, flatulence, headache when sleeping too long, dark circles under the eyes, toxicity
L2	Hip	Cecum	Digestive complaints: 1-2 hours after eating, abdominal cramps
L3	Leg	Endocrine Glands: Thyroid Pancreas, Liver, Adrenals	See organs' primary subluxation sites: C4, C5, C7, T6, T8
L4	Knee	Colon	Bowel problems, coated tongue, headaches
L5	Ankle	Prostate or Uterus	Prostate problems, dysmenorrhea, PMS
Sacrum	Foot	Reproductive Organs	Reproductive disorders
Coccyx	Toe	Overall tone of the nervous system	PMS, migraine, compulsive disorders, dysmenorrhea, impotence, infertility, dyslexia, chronic depression, vertigo, epilepsy, ADHD, sensitivity to light

> *There are 310 mechanical movements known to man, and all are modifications of those found in the human body. In this machine are all the levers, joints, pulleys, pumps, pipes, wheels and axles, ball and sockets, beams, trusses, buffers, arches, columns, cables and supports known to science. Man's best mechanical works are but adaptations of the processes found in the human body. Why not learn something of the use and of the disease of these mechanical movements? Why not use as good judgment in adjusting this piece of machinery as we do the inanimate?*
>
> B.J. Palmer, DC, PhC

The Nervous System

Most people know that chiropractic has something to do with the back, or the spine, but are vague about the details. The truth is the only reason doctors of chiropractic are remotely interested in the spine is because of what it is designed to protect – the nerve system.

The nerve system is made up of the brain, the spinal cord and the nerves that branch off of the cord. Your spinal bones surround and protect the spinal cord and nerves, just as the skull protects the brain. When the bones of the spine shift out of alignment, they no longer protect the nerve system, they are actually interfering with and damaging it. This causes distorted messages to be sent

to the brain, reducing the self-healing and self-regulating capacity. This distortion is much more than mere misalignment, it's actually an *interference* to your nerve system.

Your nerve system is what runs you. It's the "Master Controller" designed to manage every cell, tissue, organ and system in your body, and that's a *big* job. There are 11 major systems in your body, such as the cardiovascular, skeletal, reproductive, digestive, muscular and immune, and so on, and they are all controlled by the nerve system.

In foetal development, the first complex structure to appear is the nerve system, and it begins in the seventh *hour* of life. The eyes don't begin until the 24th *day*, and the heart on the 36th day, so your nerve system is supreme. It's like the conductor of the orchestra, and without it nothing else works – there's no music, so to speak. Without a smoothly functioning nervous system you would not *be*, and when it is impaired, so are *you*.

The spine and skull are designed to provide structural support, resist gravity and most importantly to house and protect the vital nervous system. If the spine were to instead interfere with the transmission of messages along the nervous system, then three types of messages would be impeded:

1. sensory nerves

2. motor/muscle nerves

3. autonomic/organ nerves.

This results in the following effects for each:

1. either pain or numbness (hypersensitivity or hyposensitivity)

2. either cramps and spasticity, or weakness and flaccidity

3. over or under function – which you may not even know about or feel.

Contrary to popular belief, the main job of the nerve system is not merely to register pain, but to run bodily functions. New research indicates that only 2–10% of your nerve system is dedicated to sensory or *feeling* nerves, so by the time you are aware of a pain or symptom you have probably been unwell for a very long time.

To successfully treat a symptom is to allow the cause of the symptom to continue.

Steven Shochat, DC

Read that again, because real wellness is all about addressing the cause, not just the symptom. By treating a symptom only and never addressing the cause of why it was there in the first place, you may later wonder why something comes back. Or perhaps it resurfaces in another area.

So what exactly is interference to your nerve system? An alteration of the bones, muscles and nerves of the spine causing compression, tension, irritation and damage to the central nerve system. This disturbance of the central nerve (the conductor) causes the organs and muscles of the body to malfunction and to heal poorly. Chiropractic doctors have a term for the distortions and misalignments that cause this interference – *subluxation*.

The derivation of the word hints at the profound philosophy of chiropractic; *sub* is Latin for "under" or "less than", while *lux* is "light" or "life". So subluxation means a condition of the body devoid of life force. Light, love, and life forces and what runs us. You know this from when people talk about a great awakening and they "see the light". It can also be referred to as "truth". Nonetheless, it is a pure energy force that is running us all.

Having subluxation means that your lifeline (spinal cord) is interfered with and damaged by a misaligned bony structure. As a result, the nerves branching off of that lifeline and your spinal cord, which is an extension of your brain, aren't giving or receiving clear messages to the rest of your body.

If you imagine a part of your spinal cord being choked and your body's electrical messages being blocked, it's easy to see how an area of the body can have less "life" in it.

All of this can be expressed in three simple, logical steps.

1. Your body is capable of self-healing and regulating, which is why a cut on the finger heals without any conscious action on your part.

2. Nothing so complex could happen at random, so something must be controlling this healing and regulation – your nervous system, comprising of the brain and spinal cord do this.

3. Something has to protect this delicate system – the skull and spine are designed for this.

So, when a subluxation stress affects the spine, it interferes with the nervous system inside it, which then interferes with the natural self-healing and regulating capacity of the body.

The 3 Principles of Chiropractic

The body is designed to self-heal and self-regulate.

1. The healing and regulating messages begin and travel along the vital nerve system (brain, spinal cord and nerve networks).

2. The spine and skull are designed to protect the delicate central nerve system.

3. Therefore, if the spine and skull interfere with the nerve system, the healing and regulating capacity of the body is reduced; that is, having a sub-optimal state of physiological function.

Vertebral subluxation or nerve system interference, causes more than just reduced health, it may damage the nervous system coordinating the harmonious interaction of your trillions of cells, which when they work together express your mind, body, spirit, emotions, strength, endurance, perceptions and character. So are they important? Yes! Do they affect your life? Absolutely! Do you have a subluxation? The only way to know is to be examined by your chiropractic doctor, because they are the only professionals in the world trained to detect and correct vertebral subluxations.

So how do they happen? Subluxations are caused by different types of stress or trauma, and any stress that your body cannot deal with at any point in time may produce spinal subluxation.

Designed to adapt to stress within certain limits, sometimes your body's best way to deal with a severe stress is a minor shutdown (subluxation), much like a blown fuse in an electrical system.

Now that you know what subluxations are and how serious they can be, you'd probably prefer to avoid them, so let's look at some of the normal life events and conditions that may result in subluxations.

4 Stressors and Causes of Subluxation

1. Physical Stressors

High heels, school bags, handbags, bumps and slips and falls, sports, lifting or carrying weights, poor ergonomics, impacts, bad sleeping habits, car accidents, and birth itself are just a few of the innumerable potential causes of subluxation. Lately, we are too sedentary. We are spending up to eight hours a day, and sometimes more, sitting or slouching with our technology. This is really dangerous behaviour over a long period of time.

Having the wrong pillow, mattress or chair can retrain your spine to sit in an unhealthy position. Heavy schoolbags have been shown to contribute to childhood scoliosis (curvature of the spine), and high heels actually change your posture, overextending the curve of the lower back and craning the head into a forward position. The trauma and tremendous pressures of the birthing process can cause subluxation in a natural or caesarean birth. We will go into detail about birth in or coming chapters.

Remember, the spine has to be strong and rigid enough to protect the sensitive spinal cord, but also flexible enough to allow you to move freely. This requires a delicate balance of forces, so it's no surprise that the system can become over-stressed, and it's easy to understand how spinal bones can shift out of alignment. Sometimes, it happens after a single jarring event, although often it is the result of months and years of unwise use of the spine – as the twig is bent, so grows the tree.

2. Emotional Stressors

Overwork, lockdown culture and conditions, financial worries, marriage and relationship challenges, health worries and challenges or concerns, traumatic events, time and deadline pressures, traffic snarls, negative friends, lack of laughter, loss of love, even changes in your environment, *all* of these things and countless can cause stress. Even childhood traumas can cause the spinal bones and/or spinal cord to move out of their normal position.

Even *remembering* a really stressful day at work can have profound affects. First your muscles begin to tense up and your shoulders rise towards your ears. Then your internal chemistry responds to the stress, you release too much adrenalin and cortisol (the fight-or-flight response) and your body goes into a defensive posture, much like a boxer. There is less blood in your brain and it moves to the extremities and muscles, so that you can run away or wrestle the "big lion" in a survival mode.

Whilst this is a clever way our bodies adapt to stress and find safety, we have evolved and do not use that adrenal response and so the stress hormones stay in our bodies. Unless you find a way to release your stress the body can, over time, become fixed in that unhealthy position by causing muscles to go into spasm. The adrenalin can actually cause an excess amount of cortisol to be released, thus leaching calcium from your very bones, which, of course, is what the spine is made of.

The entire digestive system is very sensitive to emotions – causing heartburn, indigestion, nausea, diarrhoea, constipation, ulcers – and it has many muscular and nerve linkages to the spine. Emotional stressors dramatically change your anatomy and physiology, so it's important to find ways to decrease and relieve emotional stress in your life. If you don't, that stress has to go somewhere, and you could end up with a subluxation. Over time, the stress and nerve system interference builds and that's when the dis-ease turns into disease. Have you ever seen a depressed person with brilliant and upright posture? No, they're hunched over, aren't they? Shoulders are rounded and the head juts forward. This is defence posture. The heart is closed and protected. Our physiology changes our chemistry and in turn, our emotional status.

3. Chemical Stressors

There are countless avenues by which chemicals enter your body. Drugs, alcohol, cigarettes, medications, pesticides, cleaning products, personal hygiene products, toxins, food additives and preservatives, car exhaust, industrial emissions, environmental factors and more can all impact your nerve system.

The potential effects are too numerous to list here, but let's look at one example. If you smoke tobacco (actively or passively), your body recognises the smoke you inhale as a toxic substance and may create a subluxation effect around the middle back (where the nerves connect to the lungs) to protect you from distress messages being transmitted to your brain and the rest of the body.

Subluxation can be a short-term intelligent coping mechanism, but if left for too long may become detrimental to your health. These stressors have been known to not only toxify your body but, as they also prime your nerve system into a constant adrenal state of fight-or-flight, can induce a state of exhaustion in the body where sickness and disease are much more likely to occur.

These are the more obvious categories of stress, and they cover such a broad range of simple living activities that it's virtually impossible to avoid them all. Our bodies can adapt to most stressors but with each one our range and capacity decreases and so does our health. To varying degrees, we experience and can be affected by any or all of them at any time in our lives.

When you see people who have been subjected to intense or prolonged stress their posture is often poor, with rounded shoulders, and their demeanour downcast and defeated. It takes a significant amount of cumulative stress to cause a person to respond and appear this way, and the effects on the mind and the body (the psyche and soma) are profound, reaching far beyond what we can see with our eyes.

4. Environmental Stressors

Believe it or not, there are also toxic stressors that are coming from our environment and, most of the time, they're out of our control. Just like emotional or chemical toxicity can impact on our nerve system, so too can the environmental toxicities.

These include electro-magnetic field (EMF) exposure – some call it "dirty electricity" – because the EMF frequency from radiation pollution can be all a bit too much for most of us. Some are even being diagnosed with Electromagnetic Hypersensitivity (EHS).

Raymond Broomhall, a barrister from Tasmania, Australia, has had much success with EHS clients who've been affected by the telco towers emitting 4G and 5G radiation. Some symptoms of EHS patients are ear ringing (tinnitus), heart palpitations and sleeplessness to name a few. I have actually never even owned a microwave and like to cook my food or heat it over a flame.

Then of course there is environmental pollution from the industries and toxins when we may be forced to use hand sanitisers which contain chemicals like triclosan which can be a hormone disruptor. Trying to avoid environmental stressors by wandering where the wi-fi is weak, going off-grid, working with someone like Ray Broomhall to make sure you're in a safe spot, removing your microwave oven and turning off tech for a good period of the day is going to do wonders. You must unplug your wi-fi from the wall. I don't even have wi-fi and often turn off my data (on my mobile phone). I wrote a fabulous book about digital detox called *Wellness Loading* if you are interested in removing your tech addiction for wellness reasons.

> ... excessive changes in the spinal cord may produce measurable changes in motor, sensory, and autonomic function. These are accentuated whenever the cord is stretched, and may be reversed, and the symptoms relieved, if stretching can be eliminated and the affected tissues are kept relaxed.

Dr Alf Breig
Neurosurgeon

David Feltoen, M. PhD. Professor of Neurobiology and Anatomy at the University of Rochester School of Medicine, recently discovered that nerve fibres go into virtually every organ of the immune system. He found that when the nerves are removed from the spleen or lymph nodes, immune responses come to a standstill.

We've seen that there are different types of stress, so it shouldn't be a surprise to learn that these different types of stress can result in correspondingly different types of subluxation. There are two types:

1. Structural Subluxation – a compression or squeezing of the nerve as it passes through the opening between the vertebrae (bones of the spine). It is commonly called a pinched nerve. This is often the result of a mechanical or physical stress from which the body could not recover.

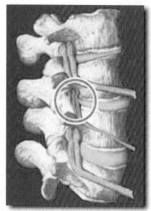

2. Facilitated Subluxation – an elongation or twisting of the spinal cord and associated nervous tissue. This is most likely associated with emotional, mental or chemical stress from which the body-mind could not recover.

Your brain is responsible for assessing changing circumstances and responding to them, and we have a great capacity to deal with stress as a part of normal, everyday life. Sometimes, these stresses exceed our normal capacity, and when that occurs, unless we change for the better and grow, we may end up expressing symptoms and disease.

While the medical community is just beginning to explore the relationship between the nerve system and the immune system, chiropractic as a profession has long been mastering this vital connection by caring for the spine and nerve system of children and adults.

As the master controller, normal nervous system function is essential to all body systems. Chiropractic adjustment restores the normal, healthy alignment and curves of the spine and removes nerve interference due to subluxations. And don't think that you will necessarily be aware of your subluxations; remember, how you *feel* is often a poor judge of your health. As with tooth decay, by the time a symptom appears many spinal problems are well advanced, and nowhere else in your body is the adage "an ounce of prevention is worth a pound of cure" so true.

So how exactly do chiropractors obtain their dramatic and sometimes seemingly miraculous results? Over many decades of research and experience, they have evolved scientific expertise and unique techniques that are unrivalled in the field.

Which Techniques Are Used?

Through its long history, many different techniques have been developed in chiropractic to restore and optimise the integrity of the spinal cord, but all use some form of adjustment to return the nerve system to peak efficiency.

An adjustment is a gentle motion introduced into the spine, intended to release a vertebral segment from its abnormal motion and/or position, thereby reducing the negative input and pressure interfering with normal nerve flow. There are more than 120 adjusting systems utilised in chiropractic today, and they include adjustments by hand, low-force techniques and adjustments using instruments.

The adjustment can range from a light comfortable pressure like the same pressure you would use to check the ripeness of a tomato, to several ounces of sustained pressure, as in the low-force systems.

The chiropractor knows that each person and spine is unique, and adapts his care accordingly – if you have been to a chiropractor before, you may have a preference for a particular technique. Spinal adjustments, regardless of which system is used, are tailored to the patient's age and spinal condition. Restoring the nutrition and normal flow of communication between your nerve system and the rest of your body allows the body to communicate, regulate and heal more effectively.

It's Not all About the Back

As promised way back in the introduction to tell you what health secrets several people who are top in their fields of work do, like tennis great Lleyton Hewitt, Arnold Schwarzenegger, speaker Anthony Robbins, Prince Harry, Mel Gibson and many other top celebrities in every field of endeavour all have in common. You can probably guess what that is by now – yes, they all have chiropractic care. In fact, some regard it so highly that they actually have their own personal chiropractor travel with them. These people became famous by being the best in the world at what they do, they are very much result-oriented and they use chiropractic because it *works*.

Chiropractic is not about the back, it's much bigger than that, and embraces a whole new way of living.

The Chiropractic Lifestyle

Chiropractic is an excellent facilitator of health, but it's even more effective when it goes hand-in-hand with the *"chiropractic lifestyle"*. This means going beyond merely having regular chiropractic care, as good as it is, to adopt an entirely new way of life based on the concept of "wellness", by living a life in which you minimise the physical, chemical, emotional and environmental challenges so that your body can heal itself more effectively.

All bodily functions are facilitated to work at their optimum through chiropractic adjustments. When you go beyond the physical to the emotional and chemical, supporting them with a cleaner and clearer nerve system, the benefits are even greater. The wellness lifestyle is taught and lived by a particular kind of chiropractor, and these practitioners are known as *wellness chiropractors*.

A Wave of New *Wellness* Chiropractors

Having introduced you to chiropractic as a profoundly powerful ancient and yet very modern approach to healthcare, we've also just revealed that there are very different *types* of chiropractors. You may be somewhat confused now if you've already been to a practitioner and not had the kind of wellness experience we're talking about.

This may have been because:

- Your chiropractor wasn't actually a chiropractor. It is possible that they weren't properly qualified and just emulated chiropractic techniques.

- Your chiropractor wasn't wellness-based and focused only on symptoms.

- Your chiropractor didn't take the time to educate you.

Times are changing, and the new surge of wellness chiropractors are focused on and dedicated to not only adjusting but also *educating* you toward optimal health.

It's important to remember:

1. This new wave of wellness chiropractors emerging within the profession encourage family care, and will take the time to educate and empower you with health knowledge.

2. These wellness chiropractors are returning to the original vision of chiropractic – not merely back care, but advancing the nerve system.

3. Wellness chiropractors know that symptoms are only 2–10% of your health. They are concerned with function and structure, with *causes* rather than symptoms.

4. Wellness chiropractors achieve excellent results because they use a powerful combination of improved techniques and new *technology.*

They will also use objectives measures of health to gauge your improvement. This may involve X-ray, EMG scan, or posture test. They want to make sure that you are changing and improving on a functional and structural level, otherwise they are judging your improvement based on the 2–10? What about the rest?

> *We are spending billions of dollars fighting disease in this country, and precious little on discovering ways to regain and maintain health – chiropractic is just that.*
>
> **Tedd Koren, DC**

Can you imagine a world where we don't just fight disease, but rather welcome it and create strength to become immune to it naturally? Your spinal health plays a huge part in our overall health and failing to address this could be your missing link to extreme wellness.

Finding Your Chiropractor

We've talked about the importance of selecting a medical doctor who is just right for you, and now I'll give you a step-by-step, easy-to-follow guide on exactly how to choose, work with, and get the most out of your chiropractor.

Treat it like a job interview where you're the boss and you want to get the best employee possible. As with any journey, the most difficult step is the first one, so if like most people your time is scarce, I recommend you start by contacting the Australian Chiropractor's Association on this toll-free number:

1800 075 003 or www.chiro.org.au and look for chiropractors in your area. You can find a good chiropractor in any country if you look up the association or check reviews. Then interview them using these guidelines:

- Are they a qualified chiropractor recognised by the Registration Board?

- Are they a member of organisations such as the Chiropractic Association?

- Are they a wellness chiropractor?

- Do they continually attend seminars or are they furthering their degree through postgraduate studies?

- What kind of diagnostic equipment will they use to measure your health? Do they take low-dose X-rays or use non-invasive EMG scans to thoroughly examine you?

- Do they see many children and families?

- Do they get referrals?

- Is their aim to educate you?

- Do they have educational seminars you can attend, or a website and social media pages with testimonials and support that you can visit for more information?

Once you've found someone who feels right for you, the next step is to make an appointment. If you have to wait a week or more to see them, don't be disheartened. You have probably left your condition unaddressed for years, so what's another week? And if you have to wait that means they probably see a lot of people, so they must have something going for them. If you are in actual discomfort, your chiropractor should be able to offer pain management advice over the phone until you can get in to see them.

In the selection of your chiropractor, it's important to know that there are different types, just as there are many varieties of medical practitioners. There are also, as with any profession, different levels of quality; there are expert and less skilled electricians, dentists, chefs, accountants, doctors, and ... chiropractors. I've introduced you to "wellness" chiropractors, so let's look at exactly how they differ from the others.

"Quick-Fix Chiropractors" vs Wellness Chiropractors

Symptom-Relief Chiropractors

These practitioners focus primarily on symptom relief, just like a standard doctor, physiotherapist or osteopath. They care for the spine by adjusting only to reduce pain, and to do so they use massage, ultrasound, traction exercises, TENS units and electric stimulation as an artificial way of relaxing muscles. A major drawback to this last approach is that unnatural electrical energy entering the cells of the body can mutate or even destroy them and, because the heart, brain and other organs work through electrical nerve impulses, these artificial currents can affect their function.

Electrical currents administered to the body have purely physical side effects of an undesirable nature. Most people who employ or promote electrical currents are either unaware of these effects, or choose to ignore them.

Dr Robert Becker, MD
Cross Currents

This type of chiropractic treatment determines your care by your symptoms and often your private healthcare insurance coverage. It may seem like a benefit that the cost and treatment time are often reduced, but in the long-term this may not be as beneficial as the cause of the disruption to your spine and nerve system remains uncorrected, and your true health is no better than before. In fact, you might even be worse off.

Your spine and nerve system are still in their improper position, but because you are no longer experiencing pain you may ignore them – they can continue to degenerate silently, allowing organs to malfunction and eventually become diseased. Covering up warning signs, in machines or bodies, only leads to further damage later on. It's much wiser to find the cause, and fix it.

There is no effect without a cause. Chiropractors adjust causes, others treat effects.

B.J. Palmer, DC, PhD

Wellness Chiropractors

Like the dental realignment of teeth through the use of braces, a certain duration of care and frequency of adjustment is essential to change the function and structure of your nerve system and your spine. To accomplish this, wellness chiropractors use very specific, highly advanced techniques in order to correct subluxations, and monitor the improvements with X-rays. Infrequent visits with non-specific manipulative techniques will make no significant or permanent changes to spinal structures, and may even cause damage.

While all doctors want their patients to be out of pain, the focus of wellness chiropractic care is to remove all nerve interference (subluxation) through a very precise program of adjustments, diet and lifestyle coaching that are unique for each individual.

The frequency and cost of care is determined by the severity of the subluxation, degeneration and structural imbalance in your body. It is *not* determined by your symptoms alone. Results are based not only on how you are feeling, but by re-examinations.

Your health doesn't care whether you have health insurance, it just knows what it needs to function properly, and cost should not be the determining factor in the correction of your subluxations. Until there is true correction and your body is completely healthy, symptoms are likely to occur again and again.

The body has an innate ability to heal itself. Western doctors are frozen in the disease-oriented model, curing disease with drugs and surgery, rather than on prevention and stimulating the body's natural healing power. Most treatments just prevent the disease from expressing itself symptomatically. Symptoms disappear but the disease actually gets worse.

Dr Andrew T. Weil
MD, Harvard University

Interactive Ways to Find Your Wellness Chiropractor

Ask Your Friends

If you have friends who share your perspective on health and wellness and who know of wellness chiropractors, then ask for a recommendation. You can ask them candid questions about the doctor, their staff, fees, availability and services offered. More importantly, your friend knows both you and the chiropractor, and may be able to tell whether your health philosophies and personalities are compatible.

Meet the Chiropractor

Make productive use of this visit. You want to know whether the practice is right for you, and whether you feel comfortable with the doctor. Some things to ask and look for are:

- Does the doctor look healthy?

- If the doctor does not live a healthy lifestyle, then this speaks volumes regarding their commitment to wellness. If the doctor appears unhealthy, then this is a concern. You want to find a doctor who "walks their talk" when it comes to health.

- Do the two of you "click"?

- Do you like each other? Does the doctor seem rushed or are they present? Do you communicate well together? It's best to avoid a doctor who seems hurried, or isn't listening well. You want a partner and a mentor in this relationship.

- Does the practice focus on vertebral subluxation and wellness?

- Some chiropractors choose to confine their practice to the mechanical treatment of back and neck pain, and this is not the wellness model.

- How you will be evaluated?

- There are modern, non-invasive instruments which allow your chiropractor to objectively evaluate the health and function of your nerve system. One is the Insight Subluxation Station™. This instrument includes a surface EMG (electromyograph) which measures the electrical activity in your muscles, and a thermal scanner that evaluates the function of your autonomic nervous system.

- The information from the EMG scan provides a baseline from the time you begin care and helps chart your progress. The reading also assists you and your chiropractor in determining how your particular physical, biochemical and psychological stresses lead to subluxations and which of them is affecting you at any given time.

- Some wellness chiropractors may carry out additional examinations, such as X-rays. These should be taken only if necessary after an examination is made and will give a clearer view of what is going on in your body from a structural and functional level.

- Although feeling good is important, your care should not be based solely on pain. As with dental cavities, high blood pressure and many other health conditions, spinal subluxations can exist without symptoms.

- Technique

- Ask the chiropractor about which technique will be used, what it entails, and make sure that it feels right to you.

- Training

- Educational and licensing requirements for doctors of chiropractic are now standardised, so make sure they are fully qualified. Additional seminar programs such as the Total Solution™ course, offered by the Chiropractic Leadership Alliance, trains full-spectrum, wellness-oriented chiropractors.

Fees

If you have a specific health issue, such as back or neck pain, your insurance may pay a portion of your chiropractor's fee. If you have no symptoms, insurance generally does not cover the cost of wellness care. If you are an Australian citizen and have a Medicare card, then you will be able to receive 5–10 visits per annum when you tell them about your headaches. The care is covered by the government, so use it.

After your examination, the chiropractor should explain to you the proposed course of care, and the fees and payment options. Many wellness chiropractors are able to offer affordable fees by eliminating the cost of billing insurance. This initial investment you make now, may save you thousands in the future.

We've spoken at some length about the power and value of chiropractic, but before we go even deeper into what it has to offer, let's look at some mainstream medical validation of the profession.

The Windsor Autopsies

Medical doctors have been publishing papers that support chiropractic theories for decades.

In 1921, chiropractic was rising in the public awareness, so Dr Henry Windsor, MD, decided to find out if its extraordinary claims had any grounding in medical fact.

He began with this question: "Chiropractic claims that by 'adjusting' vertebrae, they can relieve stomach troubles, ulcers, menstrual cramps, thyroid conditions, kidney disease, constipation, heart disease, lung and other diseases – but how?"

Dr Windsor conducted autopsies to determine if there was any connection between minor distortions of the vertebra and diseased organs, or whether the two were entirely independent of each other. In a series of three studies, he performed autopsies and dissected a total of 75 human and 72 cat cadavers to see whether or not an unhealthy spine could affect internal organs.

Dr Windsor carefully examined any diseased organs, the nerves that supplied them, and the vertebrae that protected those nerves. In his subjects he found 221 structures, other than the spine, to be diseased. He then followed their nerve pathways, and found that 212 of them could be traced directly back to a distorted or misaligned vertebra. This means that in *96%* of the instances, nerves that supplied a diseased organ came from a damaged vertebra.

He also found nine diseased organs which were fed by undamaged vertebrae, but they could also have been impacted by the spinal distortions because, as Dr Windsor stated, "the nerves entering and leaving the cord traveled up or down the cord for a few segments, thus accounting for all the apparent discrepancies." He was astonished to conclude that there was a nearly 100% correlation between minor curvatures of the spine and diseases of the internal organs. His results were published in the *Medical Times* in 1921, and they prove the importance of proper spinal alignment for overall health.

Some will say that health is a belief system. However, with chiropractic, whether you believe it or not, taking pressure off the nerve system will in turn provide a clearer message from brain to body and will make you function better, whether you believe in it or not.

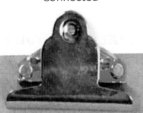

Dr Windsor's Findings

Heart Disease: All 20 cases of heart and pericardium conditions had the upper five thoracic vertebrae (T1–5) misaligned.

Lung Disease: All 26 cases of lung disease had spinal misalignments in the upper thoracic area (T1–5).

Stomach Disease: All 9 cases of stomach disease had spinal misalignments in the mid-thoracic area (T5–9).

Liver Disease: All 13 cases of liver disease had spinal misalignments in the mid-thoracic area (T5–9).

Gallbladder: All 5 cases of gallstone disease had spinal misalignments in the mid-thoracic area (T5–9).

Pancreas: All 3 cases of pancreatic disease had spinal misalignments in the mid-thoracic area (T5–9).

Spleen: All 11 cases of spleen disease had spinal misalignments in the mid-thoracic area (T5–9).

Kidney: All 17 cases of kidney disease were out of alignment in the lower thoracic area (T10–12).

Prostate and Bladder Disease: All 8 cases of prostate and bladder disease had the lumbar vertebrae misaligned (L1–3).

Uterus: The two cases of uterine conditions had the second lumbar misaligned (L2).

Chiropractic Care May Help You Reverse the Ageing Process

How Do We Age?

Each of us is made up of about 100 trillion cells, and these cells are constantly replacing themselves with new ones. The process works like making a photocopy of a photocopy of a photocopy, and just as with photocopies, each subsequent copy loses resolution – the DNA in the new cells isn't quite as good as the original. Our body works tirelessly to fix that, but eventually the quality of the new cells being produced starts to decrease – we know this process as ageing.

What is DNA?

It is the building block containing the **genetic** instructions for the **development** and function of living things.

All known cellular life and some viruses contain DNA. The main role of DNA is long-term storage of information. It is often compared to a blueprint, since it contains the instructions to construct other components of the cell, such as proteins and RNA molecules. The DNA segments that carry genetic information are called *genes*, but other DNA sequences have structural purposes, or are involved in regulating the expression of genetic information.

How Does Chiropractic Fit In?

New research shows that chiropractic care boosts important chemicals in the DNA repair process to levels higher than those in non-chiropractic people. The research also shows that no matter how old or young the person is, whether male or female, whether they take vitamin supplements or not, after two or more years of chiropractic care their *DNA repair improved.*

What Does This Mean for You?

Many diseases have a genetic component. Cancer, for example, occurs when cell division goes wrong. By more effectively reducing and repairing the mistakes that happen in cell division, chiropractic might help reduce the likelihood of you and your family developing genetically influenced diseases.

While other professions are concerned with changing the environment to suit the weakened body, chiropractic is concerned with strengthening the body to suit the environment.

B.J. Palmer, DC, PhC

Dr Bruce Lipton, PhD., trained in the philosophy and practice of allopathic medicine, is a teacher and researcher at a number of acclaimed academic institutions, including The University of Virginia, The University of Wisconsin School of Medicine, Stanford University School of Medicine, The University of Puerto Rico School of Medicine, and Penn State University. He has this to say about the nature of chiropractic and how it differs from the conventional medical/allopathic model:

"While I wholeheartedly endorse allopathic medicine in dealing with trauma or the exchanging of bodily parts, I have come to realise that preventative medicine, in the form of good healthcare, is not forthcoming from a health modality that perceives us as frail biochemical robots programmed by genes. In contrast, the philosophy of chiropractic honours the "driver", the spirit that controls the physiology. By recognising the role of the nervous system over the operation of the body, as well as the impact of our education in the unfoldment of health, chiropractic offers us profound, non-pharmacological insight into how to live a healthy and happy life."

Chiropractic is More than Complementary or Alternative

As you understand more of what chiropractic really is, you will realise that it is not a *substitute* for anything. What would we be substituting it for? Nothing – right? One of the principles it's based upon is that "the power that made the body can heal the body", and chiropractic is unique in its ability to help people tap into that power.

Other professions have tried to reproduce its results by emulating the technique, but it's the exact knowledge and extraordinary *intent* that makes chiropractic supreme.

Recent studies show that even minor positive changes in diet and exercise can have a profound impact on health, but those effects are insignificant compared to what can occur when the directing nervous system is enabled to operate as it was designed to do. Other healing modalities are certainly effective and beneficial in the treatment of symptoms and pain relief, but that is merely the first step towards better function, not a measure of health.

The true power of chiropractic lies in the life-changing, cell-transforming and rejuvenating benefits only available when the practitioner and patient are focused on genuine healing. DNA research done over a 3- to 5-year period shows that the longer the chiropractic care, the more profound the changes.

This is by far, my best secret for slowing the ageing process. I have been getting chiropractic check-ups for 20 years now.

Chiropractic is not just an injury-management strategy, it addresses causes, not just symptoms, because health is about *function*, not feeling.

Muscles are a *reactive*, not an active tissue, which means they don't have a mind of their own – nerves tell them what to do.

They don't go into spasm or become limp for no reason, the impaired nerves cause them to behave in that way.

If you are experiencing muscle pain, spasm, or flaccidity, your spine and nerve system may be damaged to a degree, and chiropractic may restore their normal healthy function. There are over 100 different techniques used to achieve these results, but the main difference between a manipulation by an untrained practitioner and a chiropractic adjustment performed by a doctor of chiropractic is the *intent*. Some techniques use no manipulation at all, but an adjustment that affects the joint within its normal range of motion. Other professions move the joint forcefully just beyond the normal range of the joint. There is a philosophy - or intent - behind the practice to remove nerve interference and allow innate healing to occur. Traditional chiropractors treat no disease but remove spinal interferences to healing.

Manipulations are a random movement of joints and do not imply specificity or the correction of a **subluxation**, and therefore are not chiropractic **adjustments**.

The purpose and intent of the chiropractic adjustment is to release nerve interference, stimulate brain function, and re-set old neurological patterns, allowing the body to return to what should be its normal state of neuro-psychosocial wellness.

Chiropractic shouldn't be compared to other professions because it isn't a treatment or cure for anything. Its intention is to improve the health of your nerve system, and everything else flows from that – oddly enough, even the healing of illnesses is viewed merely as a beneficial side effect.

Chiropractic is not an *alternative* to anything, it is a comprehensive, fundamental health and wellness care.

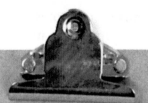

True Story

A friend once rushed up to me and said excitedly, "My osteopath is amazing! I couldn't move my neck at all this morning, and after just one visit I'm completely freed up. Look at me now!" As she turned her head from side to side, it was obvious that her osteopath had done an amazing job to restore her mobility and relieve her pain.

There are many professions that can achieve such results, and if pain relief and mobility were all she wanted, then that was an excellent non-invasive path to take.

But if you want true holistic health, remember the World Health Organisation definition – it's not about just the removal of symptoms or disease, but achieving optimal wellbeing. Osteopathic care did an amazing thing for her because it was natural and helped the pain go.

It just isn't wellness chiropractic that addresses the nerve system. Failing to address the structure and function of the spine that allowed the condition to arise in the first place is like waiting for a relapse but hoping for the best. This is by no means a criticism of her osteopath's work; for many people pain relief is the goal and he did it brilliantly. But if you are looking for genuine wellness and optimal health, then there is another option available – wellness chiropractic.

Dispelling the Myths

Myth 1: Doctors don't always tell you about chiropractic because it's "alternative", not scientific.

Chiropractic is a double science degree at university level. It has been recognised by the Government Registration Board for over 25 years. How much more scientific do you want to get?

Myth 2: There is not enough chiropractic research/evidence to support its claims.

There are millions of case studies from all over the world, and there are current research studies into how chiropractic influences DNA repair. There is also research done by doctors whose conclusions support chiropractic claims and practices, such as Dr Henry Windsor, MD, and Dr Bruce Lipton, PhD, among countless others.

Myth 3: Chiropractic is dangerous.

Statistically, chiropractic is *250 times* safer than any over-the-counter anti-inflammatory, which are prescribed and taken in millions of doses annually, without a second thought. The number one cause of death in the western world is iatrogenesis – medical error. Chiropractic is safe, gentle, scientific and effective.

Myth 4: A chiropractor should heal my condition in one treatment or they aren't doing a good job.

It may take time for healing to occur, as the nerve system starts to adapt and learn new strategies to release old patterns of tension. Most people only begin to seek wellness chiropractic care in their 30s for what may have been lifelong conditions. A quick fix for a long-term problem is no fix at all; in fact, it's usually a formula for relapse.

Move It or Lose It

Okay, so chiropractors are highly trained and extremely skilled at restoring your nervous system to its optimal capacity, but all along we've been telling you about the importance of taking responsibility for your own health and not just handing it over to professionals to clean up after you. So, what can you do to help yourself?

Train! Move! Exercise! You've heard it a thousand times before, but now I'm going to give you some reasons to do it that go far beyond mere weight control and being able to climb stairs without puffing.

The secret benefit of exercise is in the *movement*. Movement is integral to our very existence. Walking, running, lifting our arms, using our arms, hands and fingers, raising our head, contracting our diaphragm and moving our lungs to breathe, the beating of our heart to send blood throughout the body, the release of hormones and endorphins and other organic chemicals into the blood stream, the flow of nutrients through cell membranes, the molecular building up and breaking down of everything we take in and utilise, and expel ... it's all movement.

Movement creates life and energy, and I've never met anyone yet who wanted *less* of that. The spinal cord is the highway along which the electrical messages that control your entire body move, and the spine protects it to make sure the road stays clear and there are no traffic jams or gridlock. It is vitally important that the spine is properly aligned and functioning so that it can move through all its normal and imperative ranges of motion. The more structurally distorted you are, the less energy you'll have for metabolism, for healing and even for thinking. So even though the spine is the *source* of the power, the nerves are the *transmitters* of this power to all your muscles and organs, and the less movement, the less power for the body to use.

Movement benefits not just your body, but your *mind* as well. Co-ordination of a host of activities including concentration, learning, emotions, motor functions (conscious muscle control), and organ functions (including immune response) are mediated almost entirely by normal movement of the spine.

Also, research by British scientists has found that as little as five minutes of brisk walking can reduce the intensity of nicotine withdrawal symptoms. The principle is that exercise stimulates production of the mood-enhancing hormone dopamine, which can in turn reduce nicotine cravings and dependence. "Dopamine works by replacing or satisfying the need for nicotine," said Ratey.

Yale University scientists published an article in the journal *Nature Medicine* stating that regular exercise affects the hippocampus, the area of the brain responsible for mood. Mouse physiology and biochemistry is remarkably similar to human (we share over 90% identical genes), and tests on mice showed that exercise activated a gene in the hippocampus called VGF, which is linked to the growth factor chemical involved in the development of new nerve cells. Tests showed that this brain activation lifts a person's mood.

Participants in a German survey who were asked to walk quickly on a treadmill for just 30 minutes a day for ten days recorded a significant drop in depression scores. Scientists are now working on a drug that mimics the effects of the VGF gene as an alternative to conventional antidepressants.

Connectivity is a crucial feature of brain development, because the neural pathways formed during the early years carry signals that allow us to process information throughout our lives.

Dixon and Shore

The spine and the brain are in constant communication, and if the supply of soma to sensory (body/sense) information going to the brain through the spinal cord is altered or stopped, the brain will eventually respond by retreating into quiescence, then hallucination and finally into a state of coma. This means that the brain does not simply *control* the body, it also requires constant stimulation and input from movement of the spine in order to function properly.

Another vital role played by spinal movement is the nutrition of the body's joints. Today, anti-inflammatories are the 16th leading cause of death, and many are turning to natural alternatives like glucosamine and chondroitin to reduce pain and support the regeneration of joints. Joint damage and degeneration result from years of misuse, but even more so from *lack* of use. The best way to regenerate a joint is to move and exercise it, and allow the spine to perform its healing work.

Loss of muscle mass is another obvious outward sign of ageing. Building muscle tissue through exercise will not only make you look and feel younger, because your skin tautens as the muscle beneath it swells, but will also help prevent osteoporosis and high blood pressure. By the time you hit your 30s, you are going to need to focus weight-bearing exercises which are great for your bones, but when I say weight-bearing, I don't necessarily mean pushing yourself to the limit every single time you exercise, and the reason lies in the dual nature of stress.

There are two types of exercise stress – **di**stress and **eu**stress.

Distress refers to the damaging effects of improper or excessive exercise, which can result in reduced athletic performance and even promote pathogenesis (disease). Just think of the triathletes whose hearts are adversely affected by prolonged competition, the joint and heart damage of heavy weight lifters, or the significant height loss due to spinal disc compaction of marathon runners. These are all examples of exercise which exceeds the body's parameters of activity without tissue damage.

Eustress describes the advantageous effects of appropriate and measured exercise resulting in growth and development. This is a positive stress because even though the heart, lungs, muscles and other tissues and organs are challenged by an increased work load, the challenge does not exceed the body's ability to function without tissue damage. There is improved oxygenation to the whole system – the lymphatic function is stimulated and waste products removed, muscle mass and bone density are increased, excess flesh is turned into energy and endorphins are released in the brain.

To maximise these benefits, proper spinal alignment, nutrition, regularity and dedication are essential. Eustress can become distress when there is misalignment, imbalance or exhaustion.

The key is to have consistent and gentle exercise which stimulates your joints and brain, flexes your spine, and keeps all your joints nourished. Even though it will definitely make you feel better physically, mentally and emotionally, the increased blood flow and oxygen supply are not truly what stimulates the brain. Research has found that it is the neurological stimulation of the pathways between moving joints and the brain (especially spinal joints) that is responsible.

Movement is *your* contribution to your health, and it's equally important to have your spine assessed regularly by a wellness chiropractor to prevent any restrictions, gross or subtle, which may impede normal movement and stimulation.

Posture

You can get as fit and flexible as you like, but if your posture is poor you won't gain the full benefits of exercise. The word posture means "carriage" or "attitude of body or mind", and it is a vital component in not only looking and feeling younger, but also in overall health and vigour.

No matter how slim you may be, your body is meant to carry load upright for 80–100 years, and your spine is designed with three elegant curves to take the weight and impact of standing and moving. These curves act like a giant spring to absorb and distribute the stresses, and when they lose form or tone, your posture, nerves and health suffer.

The spinal curves are made up of 24 interlocking bones called *vertebra* – 7 *cervical* vertebrae (neck), 12 *thoracic* vertebrae (mid-back) and 5 *lumbar* vertebrae (lower back), which surround and protect your precious spinal cord. Your chiropractor makes sure that each one of them is properly aligned and integrated so that there is no impingement upon delicate nerve tissue, and you can stand tall.

Poor posture is not only unhealthy, it's an ageing effect that can be interpreted as unattractive – it can make a woman's breasts or man's chest appear smaller, the stomach larger and your body shorter.

Correct posture of the neck means that from the side view, the centre of your ear should be in line with the middle of your shoulder. The further forward your ear, the more distorted your cervical curve. Due to the combined effects of ageing and physical, chemical, emotional and environmental stressors, we can lose that curve – under stress the body goes into a defence posture, our shoulders tense and our neck cranes forward.

The body interprets that posture itself as a sign of danger and releases a cocktail of chemicals, including one called adrenalin. Now, in genuine situations of danger, adrenalin is excellent. It increases the heart and respiration rate, dilates the pupils to improve vision, floods the bloodstream and makes the muscles stronger, speeds up reaction time and reduces pain response – you're ready to fight or take flight, whichever best insures your survival.

In the act of fighting or fleeing, the body would use up the adrenalin and then return to normal, but without a real threat there is no action and it remains in your system for much longer, speeding up your systems and wearing you out.

Unless you use up the adrenalin by exercising or changing your crisis posture by a conscious act of will (which is hard to do, and even harder to maintain), you can set up a negative feedback system where the response to a non-existent stress is itself stressful, and release floods of stressful and ageing chemicals daily. Then no matter how hard you try to remain positive and young, the wrong signals are being sent to your brain, and you can become locked into that unnatural and unhealthy attitude of body and mind – the definition of poor posture.

When I share this message with people, I'm often asked, "If it's so important, what is the best way to improve or maintain good posture?" Although exercise of the back muscles is very important, many of them are unconsciously, automatically controlled by the cerebellum, so in this case exercise has minimal effect.

The deepest muscles throughout the spine (together called the intrinsic layer) extend from one vertebra to the next, making them completely dependent on joint motion and reflexive control from the cerebellum. With the best will in the world, you can't exercise these muscles yourself. Therefore, maintaining appropriate joint motion through regular chiropractic care (with all the flow-on effects to the brain and the rest of the body) is necessary for correct posture.

Even though there are limitations, chiropractic is able to improve posture, increase muscular strength and endurance, regenerate nerves and tissues and bones, reduce stress and increase energy.

A skilled wellness chiropractor can restore the natural curves to your spine, help your body come out of its habitual crisis posture and change your biochemical mix. At the very least, they will prevent unwelcome conditions from becoming worse, and improve your quality of life and, by the way, you may even grow a couple of centimetres taller.

People aren't living to get adjusted; they get adjusted so they can live!

William D. Esteb
Author and Chiropractic Advocate

We've just discussed the critical importance of your cervical (neck) curve, now we'll show you how to improve it. To be the best you can be, do these exercises when you are sitting at your office and desk, daily:

Neck & Shoulder Exercises

Shoulder Mobility

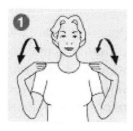

Slowly roll shoulders forward 5 times, relax for a count of 5, then roll backwards 5 times.

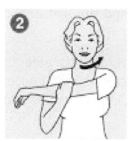

Place one arm across other shoulder and gently pull elbow across chest. Turn head to opposite side. Hold for a count of 5. Repeat for each side 5 times. Tuck your chin in and back, not up. This way you're helping to restore the backward curve in the neck. Your aim is to have the ears in line with the shoulders whilst looking straight ahead, not over your head.

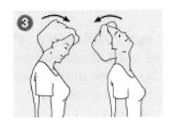

Forward and Backward

Gently tuck the chin in to stretch the muscles at the base of the skull. Remember to keep the ears in line with the shoulders. Hold for a count of 5. Relax for a count of 5. Breathe into the stomach and explained up to the chest. Relax shoulders down.
Gently bend neck forward for a count of 5.
Return to straight and relax for a count of 5. Repeat routine 5 times.

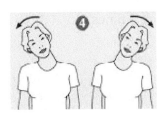

Side Bends

Looking straight ahead, gently lower one ear to the shoulder. Hold for a count of 5. Relax for 5 counts. Repeat routine 5 times.

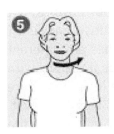

Turning Your Head

Comfortably turn neck to look over shoulder.
Hold for a count of 5.
Relax for a count of 5.
Repeat each side 5 times.

Neck Strength

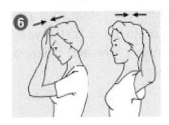

Look straight ahead.
Very gently push forehead against hand so muscles tighten without neck moving. Hold for a count of 10. Relax for a count of 5. Repeat for backward.

Sideways

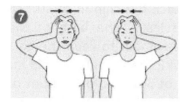 Look straight ahead. Very gently push side of head against hand so muscles tighten without neck moving. Hold for a count of 10.
Relax for a count of 5.
Repeat for each side 5 times.

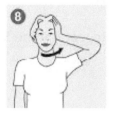 Turn eyes to one side and try to gently turn head against hand so muscles tighten without neck moving. Hold for a count of 10.
Relax for a count of 5.
Repeat for each side 5 times.

Daily Postural Exercises and Neurological Stretches

These are not designed to treat or correct your posture, but will help prevent a loss of upper cervical lordosis and assist your spine to move well. Neurological stretches are different to other stretches you may be used to. If you do this along with chiropractic care, you may be able to restore healthy posture and possibly structural changes. Pulling your chin back first, without looking up, allows the ears to sit more in line with the shoulders, which is where they are meant to be.

This allows for the perfect tension in the spinal cord, If the neck is too far forward, you are stretching the spinal cord and there will be distorted signals from the brain to the rest of your body. These exercises will help better nerve flow and create a healthier tension in your lifeline: your spine!

Exercise 1

Stand with feet hip width apart and knee bent so that your legs are in a right angle. Engage your core and press your body back against the wall or tree, allowing the back of the head to also sit flat against the surface.

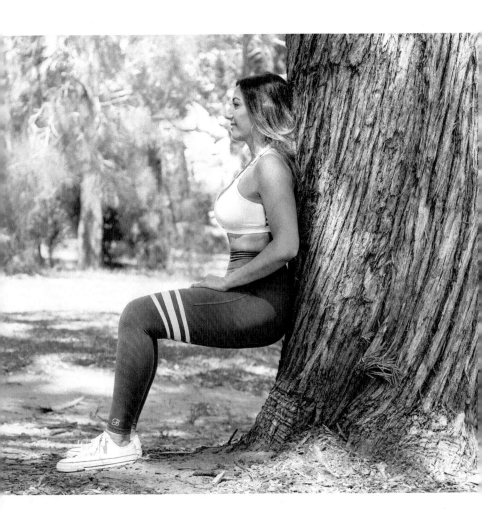

Exercise 2

Lying on the floor, take a foam roller or rolled up towel, and place it underneath your shoulder blades. Keep your knees bent. Arch over the roller with arms outstretched. Breathe into the stomach and relax the shoulders.

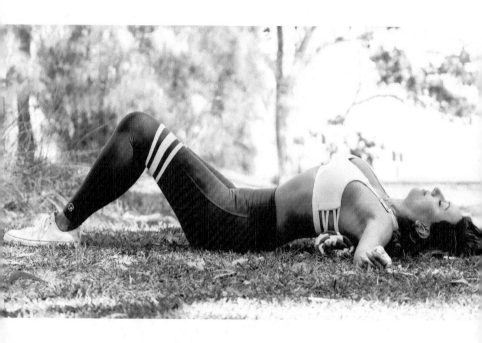

Do this for one minute a day and work your way up to two or three minutes. Roll over on to your side to get up and do this slowly.

Exercise 3

This cat stretch is to be done with feet together and knees apart. Reach forward and lengthen your spine, with your chest to the floor. Press the pelvis back and keep the chest and back flat. Take slow, deep breaths and hold for 30 seconds.

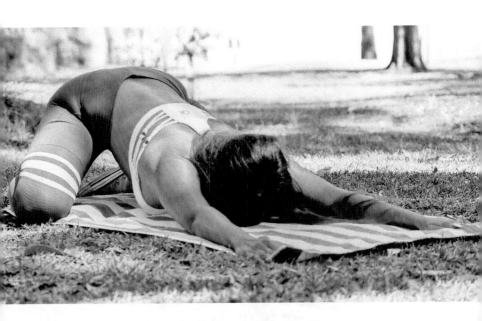

Exercise 4

This heart opener stretch is for advanced movers. Take your heels or ankles and push the pelvis forward. Squeeze the buttocks and press the chest open and up to the sky. Breathe slow and deep and on each exhale, relax the shoulders and let the neck feel loose as you arch back. Try this for 3-5 breathes before slowly coming out of the stretch.

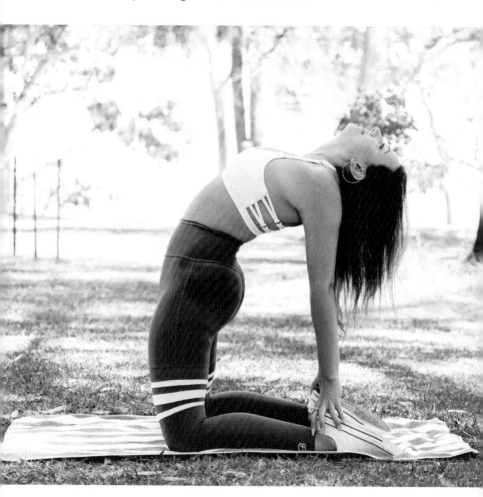

Caution: Please do all exercises *gently*. If you have any difficulty; call your chiropractor for advice.

Tips to Create a Safer and More Productive Office

Most jobs today dictate a more sedentary lifestyle as we are forced to work from home or choose to work more and more with our minds and less with our bodies.

Many laptop lifestyle workers spend long hours confined to small spaces in fixed positions, with only limited movement – sitting at a desk, keyboarding and using the telephone – and because we were designed to move, this has major health repercussions.

Repeating the same tasks hundreds of times each day places tremendous strain on our muscles, tendons, ligaments and joints, and improper design and set-up of office space can compound these daily stresses and lead to repetitive strain injuries (RSI).

RSI incidents have skyrocketed in the last three decades due to the increasing reliance on workplace technology. Health Canada has estimated that musculo-skeletal disorders, including back pain, cost the country $16.4 billion in combined direct (treatment and rehabilitation) and indirect (lost productivity) costs.

A new field known as *ergonomics* has emerged in response to these huge and rapidly increasing injuries and costs. Ergonomics is the study of workplace equipment design and arrangement, aimed at ensuring that workers can perform safely and efficiently in their work environment, and it only takes a few simple changes to make your job easier, safer and more productive.

The Keyboard

Position it above your lap.Ensure that you can type with your arms relaxed and elbows close to your body, with those elbows bent at 90 degrees, and your wrists level. Some will buy a keyboard so that your screen can remain eye level, and arms at the correct position.

The Computer Monitor

Position it directly in front of you.

Keep it free of dirt and smudges, to create less glare.

Don't have the computer screen too low. It should be at eye level or even above to maintain the natural "banana-bend" backward curve in your neck.

Constant focus causes eyestrain. Allow the muscles in your eyes to relax by taking a 20 second break every 20 minutes, and gaze at an object 20 feet away from you.

The Mouse

If you use a mouse, be aware. Some people have an unconscious vice-like grip on the mouse, as if it's alive and trying to get away. Try using a light grip, and you'll do more with less strain.

When you move the mouse, try to move your arm from the elbow rather than the wrist.

The Phone

I prefer to use the loud speaker function but if you do hold the phone up to your face, use your hand to support the telephone against your ear.

Alternate ears frequently.

Never cradle the phone between your ear and shoulder to keep it in place whilst you do something else with your hands. Some use ear pods, but the radiation energy in a concentrated form to your ear has been something that many have questioned.

The Chair

Sit upright, with your bottom against the back of the chair.

For extra support and comfort, you can purchase a lumbar roll or roll up a towel and place it against the arch of your back.

Your chair's height should be adjusted so that your knees are bent at a 90–100° angle, with your feet touching the floor. Lots of chair options are now available and you might even want to sit on a fit ball. Make sure it is the right size for you though, with the legs at a right angle, just like a chair set up.

Spending a few moments to make simple ergonomic changes to your work environment will improve your comfort and productivity. At the end of the day you will also feel much less tired and stiff, both physically and mentally, and have more energy for the things *you* want to do.

Are We Having an Awakening or Turning to G.O.D. in Healing Modalities?

Okay, so far in this chapter we've covered a lot of ground. We've explored the history and purpose of chiropractic, the role of the spine and nerve system, the causes and effects of subluxation, the chiropractic lifestyle and how to choose a wellness chiropractor, some medical proofs, the effects of chiropractic on ageing and DNA, the health importance of movement and ergonomics and posture and sleep, and even how to choose your bed and pillow.

Now I'd like to go a little deeper and address the profound *philosophy* that underlies all this practical work. I am not religious and have always said that "love" is my religion. My son tells me it isn't a religion, but I know that love heals all and that time is all we have and love is all that is real. Healing love, is unlike beliefs we may have been conditioned to believe, like the unconditional love from parents even with their acts of smacking or punishing us; told us it was out of love. Real love is gentle and kind or patient. It is a warm place to put your head without judgement and to heal in that safe space. Whatever your beliefs, you will at some point start to believe in an energy that is greater than us.

More than half of the world's population belongs to an organised faith, over 90% of the people on earth believes in life after death and around 85% believe in someone or something that created or is responsible for us.

The names they give it are almost as numerous as the believers themselves: God, Jesus, Buddha, Allah, Jehovah, Spirit, Divine Love, The Great Unknown, The Laws of Physics, Light, Universal Principles, and some scientists today are calling it Universal Intelligence. Its name and form and nature vary around the world; but the fact is that the vast majority of us believe in a higher power.

Whatever they call it, from primitive hunter-gatherers to urban sophisticates, from stone-circle builders to cathedral architects, from religious fundamentalists to scientific materialists, they are all describing the same thing – some force or being or principle that was here before we first appeared, will be here long after we are dust and gives order and structure and meaning to our lives.

Why have humans, throughout recorded history and in every culture that has ever existed, believed in this higher principle? And why on earth are we bringing it up now in a book on healing and chiropractic? Well, there is a reason.

You've come with me on this journey so far, and now let's explore a little further. You may have noticed the full stop or period in between each letter of the word "G.O.D.". It wasn't a mistake. Let's start with probabilities.

Scientists have estimated the odds of free-existing proteins arranging themselves by mere chance into the amino acids that form the basic building blocks of life, and they came up with the figure of 70 billion to one. *70 billion to one*, and that's just for amino acids, to say nothing of life itself which is infinitely more complex and extraordinary. This means that with a near-zero probability, the evolution of life by chance can be dismissed – it just didn't happen that way. And if it hasn't happened by chance, the only other alternative is by design or intent.

Design or intent, by definition, imply a designer or intender, and that requires an *intelligence*. To design on such a profound scale, this intelligence must be even more vast than its creation.

This intelligence manifests itself all around us in miracles that we have come to take for granted simply because there are so many of them. From the simple blossoming of a flower or a tiny seed becoming a mighty tree, to the miracle of life in millions of different forms springing from the combination of a single male spermatozoa and a female egg, from the spinning of the electron, to the mathematically precise orbit of the earth around the sun and the revolution of the solar system around the Milky Way galaxy – it's all miraculous design. Just ask an astronomer or astrologer. They will love to talk about it for hours.

You may have felt this intelligence inside your own body as an awakening or an uplifting of your "spirit" as we become more aware of the world and universe around us. We have felt affected by the full moon, or some say they are affected by Mercury in retrograde. You may have felt the connection when you walked along a beach with your dog, listened to the rain in the trees, gazed into your partner's eyes, or held a newborn baby in your arms. This spirit is also in the joy or laughter we share with friends and loved ones, or the helping hand that appears when we feel most alone and abandoned. It's a powerful all-pervading force which, at some time and in some way, touches every life.

And this spirit manifests inside us physically as well. Six trillion chemical reactions per cell per second do not happen by chance. The regulated renewal of epithelial cells (which line your gastro-intestinal tract) and skin cells every five days, and red blood cells every 120 days, are not random events – something is controlling all of these unconscious processes, and it certainly isn't *you*.

The nervous system is in charge of all the other systems of the body, but what is running the nervous system? What allows it to function so brilliantly? Chiropractic calls the guiding principle of the nervous system "innate intelligence", and it is the personal manifestation of the powerful creative force we have termed G.O.D. – or the Grand Organising Design. Just like the planet we live in is highly organised, so too are our bodies and they are certainly designed to heal and to evolve. How divine is that? Many of my Australian friends have been selling the word "divine" as "devine". They pronounce it this way too. However, I am a lover of language and I would like to remind you that it is "divine" because it comes from the word "divinity'. And yes, indeed our bodies and connection to the planet is divine and sheer divinity. We must honour this connection.

Modern science is now beginning to embrace the concept of a vast external universal force or intelligence that runs the universe and us. But there is also an innate intelligence within each of us that allows us to exist and is in control of all our unconscious functions. The fact that we continue to live and thrive is due to the unconscious competence of our nervous system, which is in turn controlled by this innate intelligence which is the expression of G.O.D. in our bodies.

You learnt earlier that while many people believe chiropractic is concerned with the spine; in fact, it only addresses the spine because of what is within it – the spinal cord. Now we're going to tell you that chiropractic only cares about the spinal cord because of what is within *it*, and that innermost secret is ... *innate intelligence*, the spark of divine (from Latin *divinus*, "to shine") light within everyone that is solely responsible for all the self-healing and self-regulation of our amazing bodies. The nervous system does an incredible job, but nerve cells in themselves are not conscious, they only do what innate intelligence tells them to do.

It's very much like with a computer; it doesn't matter how much RAM (capacity) it has if there's no electricity (innate intelligence) to run it and no one to use it (you). Neither computers nor electricity came from nothing, they need a designer to create them. But there would be no point in *either* without people to use them – which is how we fit into this vast cosmic life design, and why we're suddenly talking about G.O.D.

To bring it full circle to chiropractic, misalignment of the spine causes nerve stress which impedes the flow of innate intelligence, which is what actually runs and heals your body. This is the power that animates the living world and allows us to continually evolve, think, digest, emote, equilibrate, feel and love. The more aligned your spine is, the easier the flow, and the greater your potential for life in every sense of the word. It is the you that you were de-signed to be, operating at your optimal capacity.

I can't do anything for what's wrong with you, nothing for your symptoms or your pain. I can only do something for what's right within you and set that free. I can do something for that perfect intelligence that is never tarnished or hurt.

Gary Dunn, DC

A few studies to take note of:

- According to scientists in the US, patients admitted to hospital with heart problems suffer fewer complications if someone prays for them.

- A 1988 study in the *Southern Medical Journal* showed that when devout believers in a higher power prayed anonymously for hospitalized heart patients, the group receiving the prayers needed less medication, and experienced less pneumonia, cardiac arrest and heart failure.

- Another interesting finding in this study was that heart patients with self-reported religious beliefs had a median survival time after surgery of 62 months. In contrast, those patients who reported themselves as non-religious had a median survival time of only 52 months.

- (Source: November 1993 issue of the Journal of the Royal Society of Medicine)

With such widespread belief and confidence in a higher power, why do so many people turn immediately to medical intervention when faced with a health challenge? How much real trust do we place in the intelligence that runs our bodies?

In times of family or financial or spiritual trouble we often turn to G.O.D. (even US bank notes are inscribed "In God We Trust"), but as soon as our health is challenged, we forget the existence of G.O.D. and look for an outside source to cure us. Most people turn to medicine because they believe that it is responsible for our improved health and increased life expectancy, but, like so much of what we accept without thinking, it is only partly true. The most profound impacts on human health and longevity have been made by the advent of clean water and sewage disposal. We have advanced the most just from better sanitation in water and sewage. As incredible beings, we don't need too much more when we understand how our bodies work to thrive.

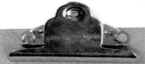

True Story

In Africa where clean water and sanitation are not widely available, the effects are devastating. One of the greatest causes of mortality is simply diarrhoea due to poor sanitation, and no medical intervention can truly address the situation (20 million children still die from it every year).

A paramedic I knew from there told me how they would administer intravenous drips to those who were chronically dehydrated, but that simply addressed the symptom while ignoring the cause. When clean water and sanitation was introduced, far fewer people became sick or died.

When given the correct environment we are healthy, because the immune system can respond to disease in a co-ordinated and intelligent manner.

A significant injury or crisis requires immediate medical attention, but disease and illness are the results of long-term processes that we ignore for so long, or treat symptomatically, that we eventually have no option but medication or surgery. Inherent trust in the body's own recuperative powers is found in such old sayings as "let nature take its course" and "feed a cold and starve a fever".

In the past when our parents took us to the doctor for a throat or ear infection, he would prescribe rest and fluids and we would get better all on our own. Today, experts say that the routine use of antibiotics against paediatric ear infections produces little health benefit while contributing to the spread of drug-resistant bacteria.

Where did the modern belief in our own helplessness come from? We believe we *might* be able to recover unaided from colds and flu, but for anything more serious we must be probed with tests, toxified with jabs and drugs and mutilated by surgery. How strange that we place chapels in schools, make religious education part of school learning, dedicate chaplains to hospitals, and make private praying areas in places of medicine, yet when faced with symptoms we ask why G.O.D. abandoned us to sickness.

We don't still quite understand that symptoms are not an indication of illness but of *health*, a sign of the body's intelligent response to heal us, so instead we call in the drugs and surgical teams because we believe that a century of modern medicine is more intelligent than the power that gives life to our every cell. We now have unquestioning "faith" that a pharmaceutical company's scientist working in another continent on a lab rat knows more about us than the intelligence inside us.

We fear what we don't understand, and don't trust what we cannot comprehend. Is this why you make a rash decision without doing research, exploring other health modalities or even just getting a second opinion? Sometimes, we also cannot understand how healing occurred, when we don't have enough studies, but Patch Adams was a medical doctor who challenged traditional treatment by dressing as a clown and healing through laughter. He created an entire medical centre and training facility based on his revolutionary approach. The results were so positive and startling that he could not treat all the people from around the world who came to see him. He didn't turn his back on traditional medicine, but used it in conjunction with the body's own healing capacity by lifting people's spirits, and they healed.

Interestingly, you don't need to believe in or even *know* about innate intelligence for it to care for and heal you. If you ask an honest scientist what light is, they'll tell you, "We have no idea. We know how to measure and use it, but as to what light actually *is*, it's beyond us." No one knows what it is, but everyone uses and benefits from it. It's the same with innate intelligence – you don't need to totally understand it, just get out of its way by creating the conditions where it can act for you and watch the results.

The magnificence of the universe far
exceeds our fantasies about it.

Carl Sagan

Some people take this concept so far as to believe that they can heal themselves through prayer alone. While the importance of spirituality in health cannot be overstated, it is unwise to rely upon it exclusively.

Appreciate that this Grand Organised Design is actually an indivisible part of you, respect that your body is both tangible (physical) and intangible (thoughts, feelings, spirit), and nourish all parts of yourself. Don't reject medical care, but be proactive and trust that through natural means your body has the capacity to heal and regulate itself, *if* you give it the chance. This is called *prevention* through *the chiropractic lifestyle*.

True health is a combination of four vital components and, like the sides of a square, all need to be present. They are emotional, chemical, physical and spiritual wellbeing, and if you do your job by taking care of these areas, it will take care of you.

Allow your G.O.D.-given intelligence to manifest healing by doing the following:

- Consume whole foods. Eat as close to nature as possible. If you want more information on nutrition, I would like to recommend my 5th book *Real Fit Food*.

- Create an optimal working nervous system through chiropractic care, and start to see one regularly.

- Exercise and move well. Having chiropractic care at the same time will allow you to be more balanced and move more evenly or freely, so the training and movement will be more enjoyable.

- Stay properly hydrated. We just don't consume enough quality water and are often chronically dehydrated.

Your body's ability to heal is greater than anyone has permitted you to believe.

Ernie Landi, DC

How to keep that "Grand Organised Designing" of your body's healing ability around for a more connected and healthier living:

- Maximise the intelligent workings of your body (G.O.D.) by removing your vertebral subluxations with a wellness chiropractor.

- Respect the fact that your body can self-heal and self-regulate when you give it the opportunity and the right environment, by removing nerve system interference.

- Reduce the physical, chemical, emotional and environmental stressors (where possible) in your life.

- Respect symptoms, they're intelligent. They are your body's way of telling you how it is responding to what you're doing to it, so listen to them.

- Don't mask symptoms with medication as a long-term health strategy.

- Don't change your environment to suit you. Allow your innate intelligence (G.O.D.) to work best suited to the environment.

Changes You Can Make

- Find a good *wellness* chiropractor.

- Get your vertebral subluxations checked by them.

- Commit to their recommendations for correction.

- Be patient and assist their work by improving your other areas of health on every level (the adjuncts) so that you fast track and support the healing.

- Ask lots of questions so you can be educated on your progress

- Respect the fact that your body is a self-healing and self-regulating organism whose control lies with the nerve system, and that healing takes time. The body also has a priority of what it wants to heal first. It's like a triage effect.

True Story

I was working in a chiropractic practice and a man would come in for care weekly for his shoulder pain. He would bring his teenage son in too after work and school on their way home.

After 6 weeks there was a re-examination conducted. During this time, objective measures of care to check on the improvement were conducted. The EMG scan showed a significant improvement in the printout. There was much less nerve system interference. However, the man was very angry. He explained that his shoulder pain was still there and that we were spending money for something that wasn't working! The changes were explained and the question asked about how he might have noticed other changes during this time. An X-ray was still due to check for regeneration but it was too soon to begin with this as X-rays don't show changes in weeks. It would be months. The man continued to show anger and his son sat quietly in the corner listening. Finally, his son piped up and said, "I have noticed changes since Dad has been getting adjusted here. He doesn't hit me and mum anymore."

The man continued with care because in this moment there was a realisation that the chiropractic care and the body's healing was not always about the symptom. That nerve system interference was being removed and what was most important was what else was going on. This was the body's way of healing first what was more important. The way he perceived the world and adapted to stress was improving. It is through our nerve system that we perceive the world, adapt to stress and co-ordinate all bodily functions. And eventually the shoulder pain went too.

And yet you ask, "Can Chiropractic cure appendicitis or the flu?" Have you more faith in a spoonful of medicine than in the power that animates the iving world?

B.J. Palmer, son of D.D. Palmer

(Founder of Chiropractic)

References

Books

Guyton, A. Textbook of Medical Physiology (Saunders).

Jensen, E. Learning With the Body in Mind, 2000 (The Brain store, Inc.).

Articles

Surrogate indication of DNA Repair in Serum After Long Term Chiropractic Intervention – A Retrospective Study.

Campbell CJ, Kent C, Banne A, Amiri A, Pero RW, JVSR Feb 18 2005, pp. 1–5.

The 14 Foundational Premises for the Scientific and Philosophical Validation of the Chiropractic Wellness Paradigm

Chestnut, J. L. 2002.

The cost of inappropriate admissions: a study of health benefits and resource utilization in a department of internal medicine.

Eriksen BO, Kristiansen IS, Nord E, Pape JF, Almdahl SM, Hensrud A, Jaeger S., J Intern Med. 1999 Oct; 246(4): 379–87.

Error in medicine

Leape LL, 1994 Dec 21;272(23):1851–7. JAMA November 26, 1997; 278(20): 1643–1645.

Spinal Loading During Circuit Weight-training and Running.

Leatt P, Reilly T, Troup J. G. British J Sports Medicine 20, 3, 119–124. (1986).

Patient, provider and hospital characteristics associated with inappropriate hospitalization.

Manning WG, Benjamin B., Am J Public Health. 1990 Oct; 80(10): 1253–6.

The Brain, The Last Frontier

Restak, R.M. (1979) (Doubleday).

Dysafferentation: a novel term to describe the neuropathophysiological effects of joint complex dysfunction. A look at likely mechanisms of symptom generation.

Seaman, D.R. JMPT 1998; 21.

The Cerebellum and Cognition.

Schmahmann, J. Int Rev Neurobiology' Vol. 41.

Inappropriate use of hospitals in a randomized trial of health insurance plans.

Sonnenberg FA, Manning WG, Goldberg GA, Bloomfield ES, Newhouse JP, Brook RH. NEJM. 1986 Nov 13; 315(20): 1259–66.

National Vital Statistics Reports.

Vol. 51, No. 5, March 14, 2003.

Sympathetic Segmental Disturbances – II. The Evidence of the Association in Dissected Cadavers of Visceral Disease with Vertebrae Abnormalities of the Same Sympathetic Segments

"Medical Times", November 1921, issue 49, pp. 267–271.

Cost and Quality of Health Care: Unnecessary Surgery.

US Congressional House Subcommittee Oversight Investigation. Washington, DC: Government Printing Office, 1976.

Job Analysis of Chiropractic, "A project report, survey analysis and summary of the practice of chiropractic within the United States"

Greeley, Colo.: The National Board of Chiropractic Examiners, 1983.

Websites

www.youngagain.com/prayer.html

www.institutveoliaenvironnement.org/en/cahiers/ sustainable-development-knowledge/education-sustainable/Fineberg.aspx

http://hcup.ahrq.gov/HCUPnet.asp

4

Nutrition is Key and Assimilation is Crucial

Tell me what you eat,
and I shall tell you what you are.

Anthelme Brillat-Savarin

A healthy body looks different on every person. You might be fit or lean, but it does not necessarily mean you're well.

Additionally, it's not just what we eat, but how well our body is able to assimilate (use) that nutrition. Just having great food is not enough and this is exactly why the previous chapters are so important.

Remember that wellness is a holistic approach to health and we must look at your nutrition in the same way too. We would take into account your genealogy and complete lifestyle and this is where we can acknowledge that there is not a "one size fits all" approach or formula to how we practice health. There are so many factors to consider.

As a certified food, lifestyle and wellness coach, I am not prescriptive with my training and even though I studied nutrition with an elective in superfoods, I prefer that you figure out what works best for you. This is because you know what is best for you, as cliched as that sounds.

Let's be consciously connected in this always, and the choices we make around eating and nourishing our bodies. We have relied too long on asking people to prescribe us a diet – just pay for the eating plan and do as you're told. I am now asking you to be inspired by these eating plans and figure it all out yourself! Here's why!

It is so much better when you empower someone with knowledge and allow them to figure it out so that they can build up self-efficacy and self-confidence for a longer-term health and nutritional plan. Once my son said to me, "Mum I know what you do now. You help people so much so that they don't need you anymore." I guess that's kind of it!

We also need to be not only varied with our nutrition – as you hear nutritionists say all the time to "eat the rainbow" – but we also need to be dynamic with our diets. What does being dynamic mean? What worked for you last year or even last week, won't necessarily work for you this week or this year.

We are constantly changing and our lives are changing so we need to change with it to suit the environment. Here is an example.

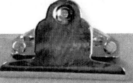

True Story

Once I was a vegetarian, and then I was a pescatarian (seafood and fish). I lived this way for 16 years. When I was in my late-30s, I was recovering from some attacks that I finally started healing from. It was a terrible time and I had tried psychology for many years but this time I chose to learn the art of self-defence with BJJ discipline (Brazilian Jiu Jitsu, which is a grappling and wrestling). I trained about 5 times a week and got to a level of competition. It was then that I started feeling like I wanted to tear my teeth into something. I literally felt carnivorous and I wanted to shred meat. I got so guilty and ashamed as a non-meat eater, and I was grappling with the thoughts of the new innate desire.

One day, one of my health practitioners explained to me that I was in a fight-or-flight mode constantly whilst training, and it made sense for my body to change the diet. I remember the day well. It took me two hours to chew through a small amount of chicken. I tried not to judge myself and I actually felt better. I saw this as intuitive eating and looked at it holistically because what I was going through emotionally was connected to how I nourished myself.

Eventually, I got stronger emotionally and I also felt like I didn't want to fight or defend myself anymore and moved towards gentler exercise like yoga. I changed my diet again and became inclined to more plant-based eating. Now, I enjoy only minimal animal protein and even though there's a myriad of reasons why some say this is better, I believe we should not judge others or ourselves, but certainly make mindful choices that are not only connected to ourselves, but also to our planet.

This is where you all can excel in 'next level' wellness, as you are acknowledging where our food comes from, how we source it, and have gratitude for it nourishing you. Call it conscious eating, mindful eating or intuitive eating, and I like to also address it as "respectful" eating.

Now, we are eating for wellness, not for calories and not for aesthetics only. Looking good is the by-product of being well. Keep this in mind always. A healthy body looks different on every person. We need to be mindful of the type of calories too, not just the calories. Therefore, when we consume nutrient-dense foods, this is more satiating than calorie-rich foods.

Satiation is how satisfied our bodies are nutritionally.

There are parts of the brain that are responsible for switching off our hunger mechanism when we are satiated on a nutritional level. This is where wellness kicks in and we use food as medicine.

The more processed our food is, the more it has been through a "process". Now let's look at the process of sugar. We now know that sugar is bad for us.

The source of sugar is actually the sugar cane. It's not just the sugar that is bad for us and our hormones, but it is the over-processed kind that is toxic because it is no longer real food.

I am telling you this because I want you to understand what you are eating and this is how you will stay inspired to eat well, when you know the process it goes through. Furthermore, we need to know how to have our bodies assimilate the quality nutrition we give it. It's no use eating the best quality biodynamic produce, if we can't absorb or use the nutrition. You may as well just be peeing it out!

Everything that lives must eat, but *what* we eat can have a tremendous effect on how, and on how *long*, we live. This chapter may add years to your life and life to your years, so let's digest it with an open mind and allow yourself time to "absorb" the startling facts about modern food practices.

Times are definitely changing, and not always for the better. In the past, we grew vegetables in our own garden and brought them straight into the house to eat. As time passed, we didn't have the land or the time for agriculture, but at least we'd help our mother cook the meals and then all sit down to eat together as a family. Today, we skip breakfast or eat it standing up, all our food is store-bought or delivered, and much of it is pre-packaged, and when families manage to eat together it's almost a special occasion.

Packaged foods are so well marketed and convenient that many live almost exclusively on "microwave meals" and "fast food". Even home-cooked meals don't have the same nutritional content as they did when soils were uncontaminated by chemicals, when "hormone free" and "no added colour, flavour, or preservatives" didn't need to be mentioned because that was simply the norm.

As our life accelerates and we invent ever more labour- and time-saving devices, the time we save just gets filled with more work, tasks and responsibilities. Paradoxically, we actually have less and less time for ourselves and our loved ones, and are less able to care for and nourish ourselves as we once did.

Although our lives have changed dramatically in the last few generations, our bodies haven't. Our genes and cells are much slower to respond to changing circumstances than our minds are, and we still have the same nutritional requirements that human beings and their ancestors have had for millions of years. When we ignore our basic needs in any area of life, there are consequences – some are minor, some are major, but there is always a price to be paid.

As times change, so should our knowledge about food. How do we get the most out of food in order to not only maximise our energy, but also improve the quality of our life and perhaps even extend it? Is it true that we can use food as medicine? Does an apple a day really keep the doctor away? And if so, what kind of apples?

Some doctors have begun educating us about good nutrition. Suddenly, an influx of nutritionists and functional medicine practitioners came into the world to educate us about food too. However, there became so many confident, complex and even contradictory 'diets' now, that many of us have become confused, or we gave up. The grapefruit diet, protein diet, Israeli army diet, Paleo diet, carbohydrate diet, water fasting, vegetarianism, veganism, FODMAP, gluten-free, no sugar, dairy-free, and countless more. And there's been a new one every week. Eat *less* meat, eat *no* meat, eat nothing *but* meat, plant based – no wonder people are confused.

I've been on a diet for two weeks, and all I've lost is two weeks.

Tottie Fields

With so many television shows, commercials, books and programs dedicated to weight loss, the focus has become solely on eating well to look better, rather than eating well to function better. But why not make informed food choices that can give you both a slimmer shape and great health?

So, if you want true health and next level wellness, even with the most brilliant working nerve system, regular exercise and a positive outlook on life, without good nutrition you won't be living a vital life. Remember that the nerve system is the bedrock of your health, and the four causes of nerve system interference are:

- physical
- emotional
- chemical
- environmental.

The best approach is to minimise negative effects in these critical areas. What you eat affects all four, and all four affect your nerves, so good nutrition is essential to nerve health and vitality.

Nutrition doesn't refer to food alone, it's also how we nourish our skin, hair, nails and teeth, and what products we use to do so. Some foods and toiletries are toxic to our system, loaded with chemicals, artificial additives and preservatives that the good they do is offset by the harm they cause. So, from the perspective of nutrition, let's look at how to keep all your systems cleaner, your mind clearer and your body free from subluxations.

Fertile Foundations

For great growth, nourishment and healing, we need the right environment. Look at the heading of this section. In order for us to be fertile to create a new life (a baby), we need to sustain our own life that is constantly regenerating, renewing and revitalising. We need a fertile environment and foundation for health to thrive. It is also just like when we need the same fertile environment in the soil for a plant to grow and thrive too.

You can't have incredible soil, but have no sunlight. You cannot also have great sunlight but no quality soil. We need both. Let's look at health in the same way. There is no one thing without another. We need it all. And this is another reason why we need diversity in health, because we need to acknowledge all the multifactorial things that contribute to our wellness, based on our lifestyle and genealogy. These all work in harmony.

We all need to be in harmony too, with each other, our planet and ourselves.

When we want to create an well environment, we need to change what is going on for us in life too.

What if what happened with 2020 was a direct reflection of how we treated ourselves and the planet? Was it calling for us to rebalance, reconnect and rediscover how to have true health? Can we look at this as an analogy for a collective consciousness reshuffling to bring back light to all living things again? Or will we stay stagnated and allow our ego to get in the way of evolution and rely on a magic cure to save us?

Dieting may work, but would not work in the long-term. A "diet" is a way of life. We cannot just get a book or "diet plan" and stick to it without holistically looking at all of the areas on why you make certain food choices. This includes lifestyle factors, belief systems, culture, what's available and your psychology.

Many who don't make positive changes to their diet are held back because of the dark energy they associate with it. They may have tried it before with no success. Or someone told them they can't do it, and maybe they don't have an environment which is supportive of it.

Like all dark energy, which is merely fear (and possibly fear of success), it wants to stay trapped in. Fear literally takes a hold of us.

When light starts to step in, dark cannot stay.

Similarly, when love steps in, fear cannot stay.

From the perspective of quantum physics, fear will always be there but will be outbalanced by the light. Fear will always be there, but balanced by the light. Where do you choose to focus your energy on?

I know this because I am a lover of language as a writer. I like to break down words and language. The way we use our words can have huge impact. The word "courage" which is what you need to combat fear, comes from the French word "le couer", which means "the heart". When you act with great heart, and love, it is acting with courage. So, fear is removed when we at in love and courage to behave from the heart.

In all my years of wellness coaching or even selling gym memberships when I first arrived to Melbourne at the age of 23, people would walk in through those gym doors wanting change. Very rarely would people walk away from me without being signed up. This was not a sales tactic. This was because I knew, deep down, the only thing holding them back from commencing that gym membership was going to be fear. Fear that they may be great, fear that if they took that leap of faith, there would be nobody there to support them, fear that when they do change, they may lose their previous lives and the people in it. They needed to be reminded that they made the choice out of love, and that I would provide certainty and remind them of why they chose to walk through those doors in the first place. They would be safe to step into their power and a new healthy world.

Now apply this message to allowing light to grow and nourish us with nutrition in order to create health.

Are you ready to take the leap of faith and step into "Next Level Wellness"? For those who already eat well, stress and mindset are the very things that may be holding you back from overall wellness, because when you are stressed, or living in a state of fear or negative thoughts, stress hormones are released and this doesn't allow for proper assimilation of nutrition.

Here's where stress or fear, and negative or dark energy, relates to the same concept of health in our bodies: when we have parasites in our guts, they can only live in a warm, damp, dark/ Candida environment. Then if we choose to get well by quitting sugar or yeast and processed carbohydrates, they know they can no longer thrice or live. They will die. In fact, the only way the parasites can then live is by dumping toxins in your gut to make you crave the very thing you are trying to give up. This is why if you have ever tried to give up sugar, it is almost impossible as you're now craving it more than ever before! Have you noticed this?

That's why you have to beat it by re-creating balance. You need to not just kill off the parasites, but rather build up the "good guys" by flooding the body with good nutrition like antioxidants. This is why we go on cold-pressed juice fasts. The cold-pressed juice is different because the motor has not heated up and killed off the enzymes. Cold pressing is mastication. It slowly presses it into juicing, keeping all enzymes intact and the antioxidant nutrition is brilliant for restoring balance.

Use this story as an analogy to not fear ill health, whether it is mental exhaustion or poor gut health. We don't have to fear "sickness", but rather understand how the body works and work with it to get back to a balanced state. Everything is connected.

Remember though, to go easy on yourself. After all, we are only human and will ebb and flow, as life is full of ups and downs.

As you can see, it's not just about food, but also the thoughts behind it and the environment we give it. Some of the greatest achievements I have ever had with my wellness coaching clients in weight loss and weight gain, came with not looking at their diet first. We took a holistic perceptive and discovered which area they believed was more important to work on.

I coached a man who had to work on his stress and work/life balance and he lost 3 kg in two weeks. I also worked with a client who had years of abuse with an eating disorder of anorexia, and we worked on self-love. She eventually checked herself in to an eating-disorder clinic. As you can see, thoroughly creating a "fertile environment" for us to feel nourished in mind, body and spirit, is crucial.

Food, Glorious Food

Now let's talk about the difference between food and excellent nutrition, because proper nutrition is an intelligent and efficient way of making sure your body stays in tiptop working order, and the benefits more than outweigh the slightly higher costs. Having said that, the more we demand quality, the more the supply goes up, which means it can be produced and provided to us at a better price. It's up to us consumers! Although health is usually not appreciated until it's gone, it is actually priceless, so it's unwise to scrimp in this area.

I always talk about making sure you are shopping for health, not value.

Most packaged foods, although cheaper, are full of preservatives and additives that have been known to adversely affect us in a number of ways, from allergies, lethargy and weight gain to Attention Deficit Disorder (ADD) and Attention Deficit Hyperactivity Disorder (ADHD). The more you can avoid these over-processed "foods", the cleaner your nerve system. So, the easiest way to reduce your intake of harmful chemicals is to eat less packaged over-processed or junk foods. We all enjoy them sometimes, but let's make that the operative word – *sometimes*.

The alternative is to eat fresh, healthy, unadulterated, whole grain foods which are readily available in markets found in every city. The choices are there, but due to time pressures, stress, habit and a lack of awareness and a lack of information, too many of us are making the wrong ones.

Organic, The New "Label"

Have you noticed how the label "organic" started to take over supermarket shelves? It refers to foods produced in environments that contain a maximum of 5% chemical residues and have no added pesticides or herbicides. So many foods, fresh or packaged, have had these chemicals exposed to them.

Many people today are no longer wishing to expose themselves and their children to what scientific research is revealing to be a widespread and growing health hazard. In fact, major chain stores now have hundreds or thousands of organic products, including pasta, juice, canned foods, cereals, milks and even eggs and meat.

There are grocers, sections of large supermarkets and stores that specialise in organic produce popping up everywhere, as increased public awareness and informed concern about the importance of nutrition has become more pronounced. It is a growing and multibillion-dollar industry for one reason only: demand. The demand for organic food has made it "the new black" or like a new high-end "label" in the food industry. But why is it? Shouldn't all our foods just be "organic"?

There was actually a time when the only food available was organic, because the chemicals didn't exist and food wasn't farmed the way it is now. People got their nutrition from food that was grown naturally and wasn't robbed of its vital minerals and nutrients. What has happened to our eating habits now?

Modern foods are so full of hormones and pesticides that the nutritional and mineral content is questionable.

Assimilation of Nutrition

It is the vitamin and mineral content that we need in order to feel full or satisfied. This is called "satiation". The micro-nutrition in food is what we need for food to not act as medicine, it is when the food actually is medicine. We will only feel satiated, or satisfied when our brains have been fed with enough nutrition. Nutrition is the nutritional content, not the calories or portion.

That part of the brain responsible for switching off the hunger mechanism when you are satiated nutritionally will only switch off when it has enough micro-nutrition, when it has been fed with whole fresh foods that may have vitamins and minerals like iron, folate, magnesium, vitamin C and zinc.

When we eat too many processed foods, we need to realise they have been through a "process". That's why they're called "processed foods". During the process of starting out as a whole food source, and becoming processed, they're stripped of their micro-nutrition and no longer have nutritional content to make you feel full or well. This is why whenever you eat "junk" or "fast" foods, you could keep going on eating them. The part of the brain responsible for switching off the hunger mechanism, never feels satiated.

Take sugar as an example. The real food source or whole food source of sugar before it is sugar is actually called "sugar cane". I remember growing up in far north Queensland, Australia and there were fields and fields of sugar cane. My mother would get so excited and asked my father to pull over to the side of the road. She would cut a piece off and sit in the car happily chewing it and then we would drive off.

It was totally satisfying and she was satiated. Why did she not need to eat the whole field? Yet, when it is a bag of candy or confectionary, we cannot stop at just one? It is highly addictive and here's why. The real food source has been through a process. The sugar cane was stripped of its nutrition and the brain never feels satiated.

Let's look at the process that the sugar cane went through to become white sugar. The first thing that happens to it is that it has its water squeezed out of it, so now it is more concentrated. If consumed like this, you're no longer hydrating. That water content helps digestion. Then, it is heated up and that process takes the nutrition out of it, like fibre, vitamin C and other vitamins and minerals that normally help you feel full. It is now raw sugar. But let's not stop there. The next part of the process is to now bleach it and make it white sugar. Then we add more chemicals to it and it becomes what? Castor sugar! But let's not even stop there. Let's put it through yet another process and it becomes what? Icing sugar! Is icing sugar real food? Have a think about it next time you eat a cup cake. I don't eat them anymore.

Now it's time to really kick the white stuff! You're sweet enough! Let's finally end this addictive relationship!

For every molecule of sugar you consume, it takes 54 molecules of magnesium to process it. Madness, right?

The WHO has taken a tough stand on the sweet thing with their statement made in January 2014, recommending sugar should account for less than 5% of what people eat per day. They also acknowledged the work of the author of *Sweet Poison*, David Gillespie, who believes that sugar consumption should be severely limited. Given that sugar is hidden in so many processed foods as a preservative or to replace the taste of fat in low-fat foods, the average Australian has been consuming 35–45 teaspoons a day. Obesity in the developing world has quadrupled since the 1980s.

Something else happened in the 1980s and that was the lies that we were fed about "low fat food". They're laden with sugar. We also need good fats to help our hormones and nerve systems work better, because they're made up of fats and cholesterol, particularly our sex hormones and the myelin sheath. The western world has deprived our bodies of essential fats (EFAs) and we have ended up with a myriad of health problems, like obesity and infertility. If low-fat worked we would all be thin but we are not!

Furthermore, sugar disrupts your hormones. The intricacy of our sex hormones is a concern when it comes to fertility. Sugar consumption will drive your insulin too high, too quickly and too briefly. You reach a sugar high and then drop fast, thus leaving you in a fight-or-flight response. It is the extended stimulation to your adrenal glands.

When sugar levels drop, your adrenals release both cortisol and adrenalin to attempt to replenish sugar levels. Eventually, this can lead to hormonal imbalance since progesterone (the hormone required for ovulation to occur) and cortisol compete for the same receptor binding sites to the body. Cortisol is the bossiest of the hormones and will always win over progesterone. Imagine this continuing over a period of time. It disrupts the entire endocrine system and leads to a disruption of all sex hormones – oestrogen, progesterone, the androgens, DHEA and testosterone for both sexes.

Sugar is inflammatory. Inflammation is simply our bodies response to damage. Be it from infection, illness or allergies, sugar is inflammatory, mostly because our bodies aren't designed to consume the quantities we see in today's western diet. And our gut goes into a frenzy trying to cope. Inflammation is a normal body response towards recovery. This is especially appropriate to women who suffer endometriosis. Most women who cut the sweet stuff out will notice substantial changes and in some instances, total recovery from endometriosis. When it comes to fertility and conception, endometriosis can be an issue as it affects the uterine lining, making implantation of the embryo difficult.

Get your body used to sugar so that you don't store it!

We are not eating real sugar so we don't allow our body to recognise it as real or whole food and therefore we store it. Start to eat the sugar that is from nature, so it is not stored as fat.

When sugar goes into the bloodstream, the blood sugar levels increase. The brain registers this increase in glucose and sends a signal down the spinal cord to the pancreas. The pancreas recognises the message and sends out insulin. The process assists with the uptake of sugar, in combination with the thyroid hormones.

Cells within the body that require sugar, but don't need insulin, like your brain for example, are already taking up sugar and will be using sugar straight away! However, this sugar needs to be in simplest form. This is glucose which can come from fructose in fruit, sucrose, galactose and all different types of sugars. They get broken down to become the glucose. The body has to be using it at a certain speed though, or it becomes toxic by storing it. The brain then malfunctions. This is what happens when someone has diabetes for example. It's when our bodies store sugar because we are not using it straight away.

In a nutshell, when you consume sugar, the brain registers that there is an increased in blood sugar and sends a message out to the pancreas to secrete insulin, and insulin helps the body use sugar. If it's not used immediately, the body will store it.

There's no use though in having the best micro-nutrients and whole food and organic diet with natural sugars if your body is not functioning well. You may as well be peeing that nutrition out, because you cannot assimilate it.

Three ways to maximise your assimilation of nutrition:

1. Have a good working nervous system. The nerve system controls the digestive system.

2. Have a heathy gut. The gut is the second brain.

3. Have balanced hormones. They're the drivers of all body functions.

Food industry adulteration and devitalisation has created the growing need for vitamins and supplements, as we just aren't getting the nutrition we require from conventional foods.

For example, huge warehouses full of imported nuts are drenched with pesticide bombs to kill the insects, so powerful that the doors must be sealed shut to prevent the poisons escaping into the atmosphere. We can't breathe it, so why would anyone think we can eat it?

Organic food is so much more appealing nutritionally, and tastes unbelievably different. It is a little more costly at the moment, but with increased demand will come the inevitable drop in price. Also keep in mind that what you are presently saving in the short-term in dollars by buying adulterated foods you are losing on your health in the long-term.

Eating organically may sound a little daunting at first, but the best way to start is with a monthly shopping trip to your local organic market which is usually very affordable. Open up your senses and give yourself time to explore this new environment. Walk around and observe the different products available, try some of the fresh fruit and vegetable juices and taste the difference, observe the different size and colour and scent and "feel" of the vital foods there.

Understand that the organic fresh produce may not always look as pretty as the waxed apples or sprayed broccoli you normally see in a supermarket – that pretty appearance is achieved only with the use of chemicals that may have the same effect on you as they did on the insects and other organisms they exterminated.

Broccoli is one of the most sprayed foods, so to make a big difference in your wellbeing you might like to start with the organic variety of this delicious vegetable. It will not only taste much better, it could end up saving you money in the long run as you appreciate it more, eat less, and require less supplementation.

Some organic foods may even surprise you with a worm lurking around in there. They may startle you, but they won't harm you, and as long as you thoroughly wash the organic food, it's fine. They're actually a guarantee of quality, because insects cannot survive in foods that have been chemically treated, so if it's good enough for the worm to eat, it's okay for you as well. You should actually be more worried that you *don't* find any worms on your normal food.

Is Organic Food Healthier for Us?

The exact nature and degree of the benefits from eating organic food have yet to be confirmed by rigorous research, but anecdotal evidence abounds, and at the very least organic foods improve health because fewer pesticides, herbicides, waxes and chemical fertilizers are used than with non-organic foods.

So, is all organic food by definition a guarantee of health and reliability? No, unfortunately even here you must be discriminating and continue to take responsibility for your own wellbeing. The meat in an organic product may be free of pesticides, but it can still be high in sugars or additives.

Just because something is "organic" does not mean it is healthy.

So let moderation be your key in both organic and non-organic foods, and let the majority of your diet consist of foods that don't come in packets. Packaged foods usually contain preservatives, and while they do preserve the food they can have the opposite effect on you.

Organic food is more natural, tastier and helps keep you away from "fast" and processed foods. Not only is it more nutritious, it reduces your intake of dubious and harmful chemicals that can have lasting negative effects on your health. Good food is not just healthy food, in many ways it can be a healing agent in itself.

If you want more "life":

- Eat foods that are alive, not packaged – fresh fruit, vegetables and foods that grow.

- When choosing more live foods in your diet, consider adding sprouts, they are new life. A sprout is the beginning of a vegetable, and will provide you with more energy as it is new and bursting with growth.

- Broccoli and potatoes are the most sprayed vegetables, so buy them as organic.

Organic varieties of fruit and vegetables will taste quite different, you may find that organic carrots or pumpkin are actually sweet. You will find the taste of these natural foods very enjoyable particularly if you detoxify yourself from coffee, cigarettes and other toxicities to remove the coating from your taste buds.

Stay away from monosodium glutamate (MSG). It is addictive, found in lots of packaged foods and can make you hungrier. It can also affect mood and make you depressed. It is highly toxic.

When juicing, the best type of juicer to use is one that squashes (masticates) the fruit or vegetable. The motor doesn't heat up like a regular juicer and kill off the essential nutrition and minerals in the food. Juicing the food in this type of blender will maximise your mineral and nutritional intake. It is commonly known as "cold pressed" juicing.

Most importantly, get rid of your microwave. As easy as it has become to prepare and heat foods this way, you may as well be throwing your good organic food away because studies have found that microwaves may destroy many of the vital nutrients. I have never owned one in my entire life. All these things add up to create a healthier body and next level wellness.

Food Is Fuel

Imagine you had a Ferrari, or perhaps you already do. Would you put water or dirt, or even regular fuel in the fuel tank? Of course not, in fact you would use only top quality high-octane fuel to get the best performance and longest life from your beautiful machine. Well, your body is a "Ferrari". It is unquestionably the most intricate and powerful vehicle on the planet, a brilliantly designed self-healing and self-regulating machine that is using everything you put in it to re-create itself every minute of the day. Putting poor quality or "junk" food in your body is exactly like putting inferior fuel into a Ferrari.

Your body is so resilient that even with the worst food, it will still produce cells and continue to function, but the long-term effects of empty, non-nutritious foods are devastating. Eventually, the body can no longer adapt or compensate, with disease and accelerated ageing as the result. It's strange that we would take more care with a man-made machine than a divinely created one, but we do. So, begin to think of your body as a Ferrari, give it only the best fuel and let it give you its best in return.

How good would it be if in the future the history of medicine reads as follows:

"Doctor, I have an earache."

2000 BC: "Here, eat this root."

1000 BC: "That root is evil, say this prayer."

1850 AD: "That prayer is superstition, drink this potion."

1940 AD: "That potion is snake oil, swallow this pill."

1985 AD: "That pill is ineffective, take this antibiotic."

2020 AD: "That antibiotic is artificial and can harm you. Here, eat this root!"

Naturopathy and Nutrition as Medicine

It has been many years no where people look for natural solutions again, and no longer want the harmful side effects of drugs and medications. They are turning to more natural means such as naturopathy, homeopathy and the use of food as medicine. As with chiropractic, naturopathy is also most effective when we don't wait for symptoms to arise but take a preventative approach to health. That's the wellness approach too, otherwise you're using naturopathy as a natural 'alternative; to medicine. This means you're still practicing medicine and it's different to practicing wellness.

Naturopathy holds that disease is a state of un-balance – a sign that the body's natural defences can't cope anymore and a signal for attention. Therefore in this philosophy, disease is not a morbid or negative function to be suppressed and fought, rather it is an attempt by your biological intelligence to alert you that something is amiss so you can take steps to restore the balance.

Naturopathy is both a logical and a *bio*logical approach – to build up general resistance and immunity, cleanse the system and produce better attitudes by using natural therapeutic measures such as detoxification, nutritional supplements, herbal and homeopathic medicines and chiropractic care to eliminate causes *and* symptoms. Naturopathy uses even more modalities than we have described, but this is enough to give you an idea of what they do and how they do it.

A Naturopath is trained in differential diagnostics and will refer patients to a medical doctor for further tests if need be. The best naturopaths will also be good educators and explain your health in a way that makes sense to you. Some excellent practitioners are also using live *blood cell analysis* and hair analysis, which employs microscopic techniques to see just how healthy you really are on a molecular level. It is important to measure improvement by something other than your symptoms alone.

Andi Lew

I went to a naturopath for a general check-up. As part of the analysis, he let me look into the microscope and I was amazed to see how inflamed and "angry" my red blood cells were, and how my immune system was repressed due to my body's dairy intolerance. I loved eating chocolate and cheeses, but all the while my body was finding those foods toxic, which affected not only my chemistry but also my emotional and physical wellness.

You don't know and can't guess how different you could be until you undergo this type of testing, and find out what your body has been trying to tell you, possibly for years! When you feel younger, you act and are younger. More importantly, you'll be healthier.

Additive Alert

Harmful chemicals aren't used only in agriculture and personal hygiene products. In the last 50 years, the use of food additives has increased to the point where it is impossible to know what we are eating. It would require countless hours to read and then decipher the tiny print on food packet labels.

According to independent studies, every year each Australian consumes over *five kilograms* of food additives. Fortunately, not all are harmful, but of 300 well-tested, supposedly safe additives, *at least 60 of these* are known to cause illness. Hyperactivity in children after eating sweet foods or drinks is not due just to the sugar, it's also the *additives* that are affecting them.

In case you thought you are immune because you avoid fast food; additives aren't found only in junk food, they are also in everyday foods like bread, margarine, biscuits and juice. Firstly, do not eat margarine. It is a man made fat and a trans fat. Margarine is like plastic and is actually black when it is manufactured and then it is dyed yellow. Read more about this in my best-seller, *Eat Fat Be Lean*.

Over 20 food additives used in Australia are banned in other countries because of serious concerns about their safety. More than 30 food additives are suspected carcinogens, where high doses have definitely caused cancer in animal studies.

Preservatives are synthetic toxins which accumulate in all your body tissues and cause breakdown of the vital fibre which keeps your skin taut. For those who would like to know more, the book *Additive Alert* by Julie Eady is a guide to safer shopping and eating. It may help you avoid reactions like asthma and other conditions like ADD, and keep your body working better.

Reading the tiny print on food packets can be tiresome and difficult, but knowing which foods are "safe" will benefit your health, keep your skin younger, and eliminate toxins from your body. Alternatively, you could just eat fresh foods which are free from additives.

The below are just some of the harmful additives you would do well to avoid.

- **Tartrazine Number 102:** Linked to hyperactivity, skin rashes, migraines, behavioural problems, thyroid problems and chromosome damage. Banned in Norway and Austria.

- **Azorubine or Carmoisine Number 122:** Suspected carcinogen, mutagen, linked to skin rashes and hyperactivity. Banned in Sweden, US, Austria and Norway.

- **Brilliant Blue Number 133:** Suspected carcinogen, linked to hyperactivity. Asthmatics should avoid. Banned in Belgium, France, Germany, Switzerland, Sweden, Austria, Norway.

- **Other Colours:** 104 quinoline yellow, 110 sunset yellow, 128 red 2G, 155 chocolate brown. Typically contained in sweets, drinks and packaged meals.

- **Preservatives 200–203:** Sorbates used in margarine, dips, cakes, toppings and some juices.

Other types of Additives' Effects: Restlessness, rashes, becoming distracted and easily bored (commonly labelled as ADD/ADHD), night terrors, anxiety and unhappiness.

Does Artificial Sweetener Really Help You to Lose Weight?

Artificial sweeteners have been promoted as the great breakthrough for weight watchers because it is practically calorie-free. However, this is misleading. Even though it has no calories, it is a chemical that your body doesn't know how to digest, and by making it harder to process foods, actually slows down your digestive system, thereby causing weight gain. As unwelcome as that is, it is actually benign compared to its many other side effects.

Aspartame, the essential ingredient in many artificial sweeteners, breaks down to phenylalanine, aspartic acid and methanol when heated, also including when within our warm bodies. The methanol is further metabolised into formaldehyde, a poison known to damage the immune and nervous system as well as cause genetic damage.

Aspartame breaks down the protective coating surrounding neurons in our brain, causing a break in the blood–brain barrier and allowing toxins to move directly into the bloodstream, with a whole cascade of destructive effects.

About 10% of the population has a tendency to multiple sclerosis (MS) but never actually develop the symptoms. These people can be pushed into full-blown MS with continual usage of products containing aspartame. Almost half of the essential elements of aspartame are toxins, making it into an excitotoxin (a substance which damages nerve cells). Research done on 1,800 rats showed that it causes cancer of the kidney and of the peripheral nerves in the head. Earlier data from the same study linked aspartame to a greater risk of leukaemia and lymphomas, even at doses very close to what is considered the acceptable daily intake for humans. Obviously, with such a list of dangerous side effects, aspartame should never be given to children.

The study concluded that consuming products containing aspartame may contribute to:

- birth defects
- brain cancer

- brain damage

- chronic fatigue

- diabetes

- dizziness

- emotional disorders

- epilepsy

- Graves' disease

- headaches

- inferior short-term memory

- Lou Gehrig's disease, also called amyotrophic lateral sclerosis ALS)

- lowered intelligence

- lowered sperm count

- migraines

- multiple sclerosis (MS)

- Parkinson's Disease symptoms

- seizures.

Another leading artificial sweetener is **saccharin**, popular because it is so much sweeter than sugar. It has been in use for longer than any other artificial sweetener, and has been subjected to the most studies on its possible effects.

When research linked it to cancer in 1977 it was not banned because there were no alternative sweeteners for diabetics at the time. The US permitted its use as long as manufacturers affixed a warning label, so in that country many products like chewing gum bear the legend: *"This product contains saccharin which has been known to cause cancer in laboratory animals."*

Cyclamate was also at one time a widely used artificial sweetener, but this chemical has been banned in the US since 1970 based upon its possible link with cancer.

Dr Joseph Mercola has dedicated his life to revealing the truth behind artificial sweeteners, and has published the results of his research in the book *Sweet Deception*. This topic deserves a whole book on its own, so if you really want to know the facts, then this is an excellent source. It will shake any blind trust you might have in the authorities overseeing what is allowed to be added and done to our food, and give you a fuller understanding of just how organisations like the US Food and Drug Administration (FDA) may be hazardous to your health.

In 1970, former FDA commissioner Charles Edwards said, "People think the FDA is protecting them. It isn't. What the FDA is doing and what the people think it's doing are different as night and day." (San Francisco Chronicle January 2, 1970). According to Edwards, the FDA not only works to protect 'pharma-business', but also actively works against good health practices and has done so for years.

While no sweetener is without controversy, artificial sweeteners can be quite damaging to our health and may cause serious illness. If you have the choice, and you *do*, its best to avoid them completely. Some people choose them because they believe an artificial sweetener is actually healthier and better for them than sugar. *It is not*. All artificial sweeteners are exactly that – artificial.

Others choose them over sugar because they believe it will help them to lose weight. But do artificial sweeteners help us fight the battle of the bulge? Absolutely not. There are *no* studies proving that diet drinks assist weight loss.

In fact, the very opposite is true. The sweetness of the drink tends to stimulate appetite, especially for more sweets. A recent study found that those who drank diet drinks had a greater likelihood of being obese and overweight than the average person, and even more than those who drank only regular soft drinks. Why? Because diet drinks trigger sugar craving.

In addition, drinking diet drinks provides a false sense of security; people feel they've "earned the right" to eat more, and can actually increase their daily calorie intake. And if all that isn't enough, diet soft drinks also trigger the body to store more fat.

All this is done in the quest to avoid sugar, but is the fear justified? A gram of sugar contains a mere four calories (a teaspoon about 15, a tablespoon 45). While overuse of sugar has its own issues, if you're going to indulge on occasion, it's much healthier to make it real.

More Sickly Sweet News About Aspartame

You're now getting an inkling of the possible dangers of regular aspartame consumption. There are countless reports and research from doctors and nutritionists who have "cured" their clients of many conditions, simply by removing aspartame from their diets.

The multibillion-dollar aspartame industry would have us believe that "aspartame kills" is an urban legend, and that it would require the consumption of 100 cans of diet soda a day for harm to come from their product. This is not true.

Their main claim is that the three components of aspartame are found in many natural foods and are therefore safe. This is like saying that carbon monoxide is safe because it contains oxygen, the same components we use to breathe.

Methanol (wood alcohol) makes up 10% of aspartame and is highly toxic – the minimum lethal dose for an adult is two teaspoons. It is found in some fruits and vegetables, but never occurs in natural foods without ethanol and pectin, its "antidotes". Ethanol and pectin prevent methanol from being metabolised into formaldehyde (embalming fluid) and formic acid (the same chemical as fire ant venom), both deadly toxins. An ethanol drip is the standard emergency room treatment for methanol poisoning. Aspartame contains no ethanol or pectin, therefore the methanol is converted to formaldehyde and formic acid in your body when you consume it.

Most foods that are labelled "low fat" or "light" will contain artificial sweetener, and again you may think you're losing weight or being healthier by eating less sugar or fat, but these chemicals slow down the digestive system and may actually make you put on weight.

The effects go beyond this. Studies show that long-term use creates an environment for blood-borne cancers, like lymphoma, to develop. Imagine, all this time we have been led to believe that we were making healthier choices when we opted for artificial sweeteners, just because they had fewer calories.

If you're diabetic, then you have good reason to seek alternative sweet sources, but choose wisely. There are many natural sweeteners that are much safer than any artificial ones, and once you reduce your sweet consumption it's likely that your cravings will also abate.

Andi Lew

My grandmother was an incredible woman. Margot (bless her) was quite proud of her figure. She loved artificial sweeteners as it was just the way you were conditioned to consume during her generation and she ate the pills for her hot drinks or foods with them most of her life. However, she eventually became riddled with lymphoma, and one day as she lay in bed I came to share with her what I had learned from my research.

English is not her first language, so I said to her very simply, "No more aspartame. It's poison. I will show you the research."

She replied, "What do you mean? I have been having it my whole life!" This was exactly my point.

Chemicals, noun: noxious substances from which modern foods are made.

Unknown

Sugar Alternatives

Stevia is made from the leaves of the South American plant *Stevia rebaudiana*. As a herb and a natural sweetener it is superior to any artificial product. Sweeter than regular sugar and with far fewer calories, it is used to sweeten tea in Japan and South America. Stevia is beneficial in balancing blood sugar, and has antimicrobial properties. Again, moderation is the key, but when such excellent herbal alternatives are available you needn't sweeten anything artificially.

Xylitol is another alternative to sugar and artificial sweeteners, and may be used safely in small amounts. Derived from the birch tree, it is widely used in chewing gums as it inhibits bacterial growth and reduces the incidence of cavities. It tastes exactly like sugar, and is especially good for diabetics and those who are hypoglycaemic.

A 1986 study verified xylitol's safety – it received the highest and safest ADI (acceptable daily intake) rating. You can purchase xylitol from health food stores and most holistic dentists to use as a sweetener in drinks and baked goods.

Coconut sugar, Rapadura sugar and monk fruit sugar are all great alternatives too. They're more natural and less processed.

A report by Felicity Lawrence in the Guardian on September 30th, 2005, further explored the controversy surrounding man-made artificial sweeteners.

> Aspartame, the artificial sweetener used in more than 6,000 food and drink products around the world, is the subject of renewed controversy this week after the results of the latest research into whether it can cause cancer.
>
> Scientists at the independent European Ramazzini Foundation for cancer research in Bologna presented new results from its long-term, large-scale study of the effect of aspartame on 1,800 rats, at its international conference on cancer and environmental sciences in Italy last week. The research centre said analysis of its latest results showed aspartame caused cancer of the kidney, and of the peripheral nerves, mainly in the head. Earlier data from the same study published in July linked aspartame to an increased risk of leukaemias and lymphomas in female lab rats "at doses very close to the acceptable daily intake for humans". ...
>
> ... The rats were studied for nearly three years, until the end of their natural lifespan; most studies last about two years. Six different dose levels were tested against a control group not given aspartame. The National Toxicology Programme of the US National Institutes of Health convened a pathology working group to provide a second opinion on the interpretation of some of the cancerous lesions observed by the Ramazzini researchers, and helped with the statistical evaluation

of data. The Italian scientists concluded that aspartame is a "multipotential carcinogen", causing a dose-related increase in leukaemias and lymphomas in female rats, and a dose-related increase in incidence of cancer and its precursors in the kidney (renal pelvis and ureter) as well as tumours in the peripheral nerves, in particular in cranial nerves. ...

... The researchers also found that while rats fed aspartame ate less food, there was no difference in weight between treated and untreated animals.

... The foundation is now planning to enlarge its study to embryonic rats and mice – work that will take several years to complete. Meanwhile, one of the authors of the study, Fiorella Belpoggi said: "In our opinion, the results of our first experiment on aspartame call for urgent reconsideration of the rules governing its use as an artificial sweetener." ...

The good news is that you needn't continue to put these destructive chemicals into your body because there are natural calorie-free alternatives. Stevia and Xylotol, derived from natural plants, provide all of the sweetening power with none of the abovementioned side effects.

If you must sweeten food and you don't have a weight issue or a hormonal problem, then your best choice is organic raw sugar or even honey in moderation, but these other plant-derived sweeteners can be used as a safe and healthy source for the natural sweetness that we all love. For a honey alternative for vegans, try rice malt syrup which is also lower GI. Then there's also coconut syrup too which is delicious on pancakes!

Moving Mercury Out – It's Fishy Business

Researchers suggest that many varieties of fish have high levels of mercury in their bodies for better insulation and to regulate their body temperature, and the bigger the fish the higher the levels of mercury they contain. Why is this so? Because the big fish eat little fish, and the more fish they eat the more mercury they are consuming. Also, most big fish prefer deeper waters which tend to be cold, so they need the higher levels of insulation which, some researchers suggest, mercury provides.

In fish it's a necessary element but in humans it is an extremely toxic substance. Tuna and flake from some fish and chip shops have high mercury levels, so pregnant women especially should avoid eating these varieties, as mercury toxicity can be very risky to the health and life of the baby. The best fish are small ones like sardines, flathead and blue grenadier.

Fish contains very high levels of nutritious enzymes and beneficial fats such as omega-3 oils, so you don't want to completely avoid it. Just eat it wisely and well. The EFAs (essential fatty acids) in foods are crucial for helping the nerve system and hormones. This is why they are called "essential" fatty acids.

Another, and indeed the most common, source of chronic exposure to mercury is the amalgam in dental fillings. While some dentists maintain that mercury is virtually inert as a filling, others in the profession, such as holistic dentists who look at the whole person and not just the disease, state categorically that it is still toxic. The key word is "virtually", because the fact is that there will always be a certain amount of molecular transfer of mercury due to wear and the acidic environment of the mouth. Despite their protestations of perfect safety, and even though it is tougher and more durable than the modern alternatives, few if any dentists use mercury fillings today.

Having your amalgam fillings removed may be a fairly costly exercise, but much less so than the long-term health effects of leaving them in your body. Dental mercury may have actually lowered your immune system and contributed to stress, depression and mood swings. Before you begin the removal process, talk to a holistic dentist who knows the appropriate herbs and natural medicines to negate the effects of the mercury. Replacing your mercury fillings with porcelain, ceramic, gold or any of the latest safe alternatives to amalgam is not just a cosmetic measure. It will have a dramatically positive impact on your health, with a more beautiful smile as a bonus. You want to avoid mercury wherever it may be, and a range of homeopathic treatments and heavy metal toxicity detoxes are available.

Dairy – Mooooving Away From Milk

It's not just vegans who are promoting "dairy free" alternatives. You only have to look at the wide variety of non-dairy milk choices available now to understand it has not just become an ethical choice to eat less cow products, but also a health choice.

Almost everyone who's a little older reading this has fond and comforting memories of pouring creamy dairy milk over cereal, or into the tall, cold glass after school. As adults we are still tempted by the delights of tasty, decadent chocolates and exotic cheeses. Beautiful models and television doctors tell us how good for us milk is, and a cosy, warm drink of milk before bed has become a tradition. Milk was our very first food, suckled from our mother's breast. Throughout life, consuming lavish amounts of dairy in the form of cheese, yoghurt, milk, butter and chocolate has become so common that it seems perfectly natural.

Dietitians insisted you need milk for calcium to build strong teeth and bones. The food pyramid we were taught in school has an entire level dedicated to dairy products as a vital part of any balanced diet, and school lunches almost always included milk and even hospital meals are the same. With such widespread acceptance, and so many experts promoting it, dairy must be good for us, right? Well, increasing numbers of studies are showing that it isn't, and we're going to see exactly why our faith in dairy may be a misplaced trust. A new wave of nutritionists and naturopaths or function medicine doctors have been educating us on healthier options, making claims it causes inflammation.

Why are so many people today eliminating dairy products from their diets altogether? Although it may sound radical to those of us raised on milk, it is an eminently viable health choice. Of all mammals, only humans continue to drink milk beyond infancy. Professional singers, actors, and speakers scrupulously avoided dairy for years to protect their throat and vocal cords, expressing that they experienced a "dairy bubble" in their throats, and the rising incidence of allergies and illness from over-consumption of this food should at least make us stop and reassess.

There are obviously two diametrically opposed camps on the subject, so who is right? Can we trust the milk industry spokesmen whose livelihoods depend on us using their product? Where should we get our information on this controversial subject, and who can we trust? Increasingly, these nutritional experts are urging caution. May I suggest that you figure out what feels right for you? We can certainly all benefit from at least minimising or trying other options.

Let's examine one of the major claims for the value and benefits of milk consumption – it's a preventive to osteoporosis.

Osteoporosis is a debilitating disease, usually of the elderly but also suffered to some degree by women going through menopause, characterised by reduced bone density. Bones become thinner and more brittle, sometimes honeycombed with hollow chambers, and can be so weakened that they break or fracture easily. A fall that would normally result in nothing more serious than a bruise can cause a broken leg, hip, shoulder or pelvis and a stay in hospital. Otherwise vital elderly people with many years of life left in them can go rapidly downhill through confinement, lack of exercise and stimulation, and exposure to hospital bacteria (iatrogenia again). This serious illness has therefore affected the quality of, and even cut short, many lives.

Bones consist mainly of calcium, and to aid in the formation and maintenance of strong bones and teeth we are told to drink cow's milk for its high calcium content. But then why do Australians (who consume so much of it) have one of the world's highest incidences of osteoporosis? And why do nations consuming the most dairy have the world's worst rates of bone density and osteoporosis? If dairy is such a good dietary source of calcium, surely the countries which consume little or none of it would suffer more bone loss – yet, strangely, they do not. Cow's milk is actually a very poor source of calcium for humans because of all the physical complications it causes.

The dairy industry spends millions of dollars advising us to drink milk to ensure healthy bones, but is there actually a calcium emergency? Does every body really need milk? Professor Walter Willet of the Harvard School of Public Health, chairman of the nutrition department, had this to say: "There is no evidence that we have a calcium emergency, as the dairy industry would have us believe. We have one of the highest calcium intakes in the world."

So is the osteoporosis epidemic in Australia, US and other first-world nations really caused by drinking too little milk? Perhaps we should look at countries where people consume even more milk than we do – Denmark, Holland, Norway and Sweden. The verdict? They have rates of osteoporosis *higher than ours*. This suggests that increased milk consumption may have the opposite effect of what we've been told by the "experts", and actually lead to higher osteoporosis rates. When it comes to bone density, the real question seems not to be how much calcium we consume in our diet, but how much calcium we prevent from leaving our bones.

This naturally brings up the question, what causes calcium to leave the bones? The answer is surprising. Regardless of how much calcium you take in, the amount your body can actually *absorb* and assimilate is what matters. Digesting any animal protein creates an acidic environment in the body. This interferes with normal organic functioning because your body has a pH level where it is most efficient.

Calcium is the opposite of acid. It's an alkaline, so in order to return to a neutral state the body turns to the nearest source of calcium and leaches it from the skeleton. The longer this situation continues, the greater the risk of osteoporotic deformation. This is a particular problem in countries where animal product consumption is high. So, osteoporosis is combatted not by increasing our dairy intake, but by reducing our meat consumption.

The American Journal of Epidemiology reported, "Consumption of dairy products ... was associated with an increased risk of hip fractures ... metabolism of dietary protein causes increased urinary excretion of calcium ... [because]... dietary protein increases production of acid in the blood which can be neutralized by calcium mobilised from the skeleton," according to the *American Journal of Clinical Nutrition*.

Decades of clever marketing slogans have convinced the public that milk is "nature's perfect food". But it is hardly perfect for 90% of Asians, 70% of Africans, 50% of Hispanics and 15% of Caucasians who may be lactose intolerant, or as we are about to learn, may be "casein" intolerant.

So, what will happen to your bones and teeth if you stop drinking milk? The majority of the world's population takes in less than half the calcium we are told we need, yet they have strong bones and healthy teeth. Cow's milk is rich in phosphorous, which can combine with calcium and prevent you from absorbing the calcium in milk, and milk protein accelerates calcium excretion from the blood through the kidney. So not only does it reduce the intake of calcium, it also increases the output, and you lose in two ways.

If you want more calcium, the best place to find it is where healthy cows should get it in the first place – *greens, leafy vegetables and grass*. Cows eat it all day every day, and we would be wise to "cut out the middleman" (or cow), and go straight to the source ourselves by eating more of these vital foods. It is possible to obtain all your daily calcium needs from dark leafy green vegetables, and the darker the better. Cooked collard greens and kale are especially good sources. You also have calcium in almonds. These food sources of calcium are more bio-available to our bodies.

Everyone wants stronger, healthier teeth and bones, which require calcium, but dairy products are not the answer.

Some excellent sources are:

- cabbage
- dark, leafy green vegetables
- almonds
- sesame seeds
- Tahini (hulled or unhulled paste, as it is made from sesame seeds)
- figs (dried or fresh)
- small fish with bones intact (e.g. anchovies and sardines).

Half the work that is done in the world is to make things appear what they are not.

E.R. Beadle

Allergies

The generalisation that cow's milk benefits "everybody" overlooks the glaring fact that milk is acknowledged by health professionals around the world as one of the most potent allergy-inducing foods. Milk is linked to a whole spectrum of children's chronic health problems, including such maladies as recurrent ear infections, constipation, sinus congestion, asthma and skin problems like acne, to name only a few. Many doctors have discovered that simply eliminating dairy products from the diet, *and taking no other action*, can relieve these conditions and improve the health of many children. In susceptible people, dairy products also appear to be immunogenic – that is, capable of triggering an auto-immune response such as Type I diabetes.

Diabetes

Several studies have linked cow's milk to diabetes in children. The exact link has yet to be traced, but it is believed that one of the constituents of milk, bovine serum albumin, may cause the immune system to turn on and destroy insulin-producing cells in those dairy-fed diabetic children.

Breast-fed infants who do not drink cow's milk are less susceptible to diabetes, and avoiding cow's milk may delay or prevent diabetes in susceptible individuals. A 2003 study of 4,701 ten- to sixteen-year-olds from eleven European countries found that cow's milk and animal-product consumption were associated with higher rates of Type 1 diabetes, when Icelandic data was excluded.

According to Diabetes Care, a publication of the American Diabetic Association, "Early cow's milk exposure may be an important determinant of subsequent Type I diabetes and may increase the risk approximately 1.5 times." That's a 150% risk increase. In adults, a flood of scientific evidence relates milk drinking to such disorders as irritable bowel syndrome and Crohn's disease, obesity, arthritis and even cancer. The hormones present in cow's milk also seem to trigger abnormal hormonal responses in humans.

Thousands of scientific articles over the past 20 years have shown that milk is in fact causing health problems such as intestinal colic, intestinal irritation, intestinal bleeding, anaemia, allergic reactions in infants and children and infections such as salmonella. More ominous is the fear of viral infection with bovine leukaemia virus or an AIDS-like virus as well as concern for childhood diabetes.

Contamination of milk by blood and white (pus) cells as well as a variety of chemicals and insecticides is also of great concern. In adults, the problems are centred more around heart disease, arthritis, allergy, sinusitis and the even more serious questions of leukaemia, lymphoma and cancer.

So, with such a dramatic list of illnesses, diseases and detrimental health effects, why on earth do we persist in consuming dairy products? Perhaps because it was our first food and we have an unconscious attachment to it? But milk is a short-term nutrient for newborns, and that's all nature intended it to be; when the time comes for weaning, young mammals are introduced to the proper food for their species. A dog mother nurses her pup for just eight weeks before teaching it to eat solid food, and though the duration of the milk-feeding time varies, all animals follow suit – except humans. The general rule is that most animals are exclusively breast-fed until they have tripled their birth weight, which in human infants occurs around the age of one year. In no mammal except humans (and the occasional domestic cat) is milk consumption prolonged beyond the weaning period.

We don't even drink human milk anyway, but have selected cow's milk as the "perfect food" for us throughout life. However, the milk of most mammals varies considerably. For example, the milk of goats, elephants, cows and camels all have very different fat, protein, sugar, and mineral compositions, and each was designed to provide optimum nutrition for the young of their respective species. Human milk is not suitable for these animals, just as their milk is not suitable for us.

How would you like to be tucked up into bed with a nice warm cup of dog's milk? No? All right then, how about a tall cold glass of cat milk on a hot afternoon? It sounds silly and even somewhat repugnant, but people who've investigated it feel the same way about cow milk. Human milk is for human infants, dog's milk for pups, cat's milk for kittens, and cow's milk for calves – period. We may have settled on the cow for its docile nature and abundant milk supply, but is it natural? Somehow, this choice seems "normal" and validated by our culture and long-standing custom, but is it really wise to drink the milk of another species?

Much of the problem stems from not just the nature of milk, but its production and *processing* as well. Modern feeding methods turn healthy milk products into allergens and carcinogens. This happens when high protein, soy-based feeds are substituted for fresh green grass, and selective breeding creates cows with abnormally large pituitary glands so that they produce three times more milk than the old-fashioned cow. On top of this genetic distortion, fifty years ago the average cow produced 2,000 pounds of milk per year, while today the top producers give 50,000 pounds. This is only possible through the wholesale administration of drugs, which find their way into the meat, milk and all the dairy foods these creatures produce.

Due to the abnormal feeds cows are now given, they also need antibiotics to keep them well. The milk is then pasteurised so that all valuable enzymes are destroyed. These enzymes are essential for milk digestion, and as the human pancreas is not always able to produce them, overstress of the pancreas may lead to diabetes and other diseases. In response to our recent obsession with body image, the dairy industry has introduced versions of milk with the normal fat reduced or removed, such as skim milk.

Selling skim milk as a "health product" is deceptive, because the butterfat is there for a good reason. Butterfat contains acids which have strong anti-carcinogenic properties. When it is removed by homogenisation, the milk is almost totally devoid of vitamin A, and without the butterfat the body cannot absorb and utilise the vitamins and minerals in the remaining water fraction of the milk. Synthetic vitamin D, a known liver toxin, is added to replace the natural vitamin D complex in butterfat.

Milk and Infants

A committee on nutrition of the American Academy of Pediatrics reported on the use of whole cow's milk in infancy: "... whole milk should not be fed to the infant in the first year of life because of its association with iron deficiency anemia (milk is so deficient in iron that an infant would have to drink an impossible 31 quarts a day to get the RDA of 15 mg), acute gastro-intestinal bleeding, and various manifestations of food allergy ... unmodified whole bovine milk should not be consumed after infancy because of the problems of lactose intolerance, its contribution to the genesis of athero-sclerosis, and its possible link to other diseases." (Pediatrics 1983: 72–253)

In an article published in *The New England Journal of Medicine* article dated July 30, 1992, Dr Benjamin Spock, possibly the best-known pediatrician in history, articulated the same thoughts and specified avoidance for the first two years of life.

> "I want to pass on the word to parents that cows' milk from the carton has definite faults for some babies. Human milk is the right one for babies. A study comparing the incidence of allergy and colic in the breast-fed infants of omnivorous and vegan mothers would be important. I haven't found such a study; it would be both important and inexpensive. And it will probably never be done."

This study stems from the Hospital for Sick Children in Toronto and from Finnish researchers. In Finland, there is "... the world's highest rate of dairy product consumption, and the world's highest rate of insulin-dependent diabetes. The disease strikes about 40 children out of every 1,000 there, contrasted with six to eight per 1,000 in the United States. Antibodies produced against the milk protein during the first year of life, the researchers speculate, also attack and destroy the pancreas in a so-called auto-immune reaction, producing diabetes in people whose genetic makeup leaves them vulnerable."

This study found that of the 142 Finnish children with newly diagnosed diabetes, everyone had at least eight times as many antibodies against the milk protein as did healthy children, which is clear evidence that these children had a raging auto-immune disorder.

Not everyone is intolerant to dairy or wants to give it up and that is completely okay. It is your choice.

So what do you have to gain though, by experimenting with the removal of dairy from your diet? Everything we've talked about, and more. Some people mourn the loss of their favourite foods as a consequence of healthier eating habits, but fear not, all is not lost. Dark organic chocolate in moderate amounts is high in anti-oxidants and is actually good for you. It's easy to replace the morning's cereal milk with almond, coconut, macadamia nut, oat or rice milk, and if you love cheese, or are lactose intolerant, you may opt for goat's cheese.

It is true that goat milk is still different from human milk, but their products have a less irritating effect on our bodies. They are less flocculent, that is, the fat occurs in much smaller globules than with cow products, and so are much more easily digested. And for those who love butter, there is no question that it is much healthier than margarine, which is produced by bubbling nitrogen through vegetable oil, with nickel as a catalyst. Not all of the nickel is recovered, so you're getting more heavy metal in your system. But even more alarming is the fact that if they continue the process a little longer the margarine turns into plastic. That's right, yummy plastic!

As for butter versus margarine, I trust cows more than chemists.

Joan Gussow

The use of bovine growth hormone (BGH) by dairy farmers to increase their milk production is a strong indictment of the safety of milk and dairy products. BGH also causes cows to have an increase in breast infections for which they must receive additional antibiotics. So aside from the initial dosages of antibiotics, the cows often receive another round to counter the effects of the drugs they are given. These accumulate in the system and again are passed into the milk that we then drink as a "healthy" product. By drinking milk, you are likely consuming significant amounts of antibiotics.

Giving up dairy isn't for everyone, for a variety of reasons, but it can be excellent for some people, and you won't know which kind you are until you try. I found it very hard to give up my beloved cheese, but only when I went for periods without it did I realise how unhealthy my body became the moment

I reintroduced it – an uncomfortable build-up of mucus was almost instantaneous.

If you find it difficult, give it a trial for several weeks only, and then re-evaluate how you feel afterwards. It will take about two weeks for dairy to completely leave your system, and eating the smallest amount will add another two weeks to the process. To be meaningful, this test should include all dairy, including skim milk and Lact-aid milk, cheese, yoghurt, chocolate and ice cream. Don't forget how many products or café-bought items have diary added too when you try this.

If you feel better after several weeks, you can then further experiment by reintroducing small amounts of one form of milk every four days, and noting the effect of each variety on your wellbeing. Most people will likely consume dairy in some form anyway, either through eating out or in processed foods, and small amounts are unlikely to cause any noticeable problems.

For babies; it is very important that they receive proper nutrition. Breast milk is best from the mother who also does not consume dairy. Goat's milk formula is also available.

I would like to suggest reading any material by Lactation Consultant Pinky McKay to learn more about breast feeding your child.

Dairy to be different

Cheese	Goat's milk feta or spreadable goat's cheese. Be sure to read the label as some goat's cheese also contains cow dairy. Hard yellow goat's cheese is rare, but are available.
Ice cream	Vegan varieties made with coconut milk, like Cocofrio, fruit icy-poles, non-dairy based sorbet.

Butter	Spreads made from flaxseed oil, olive oil on bread. For cooking, cold-pressed coconut oil.
Cream	Coconut milk.
Yoghurt	Avoid soy yoghurts as they contain high levels of phytoestrogens. You should find an alternative snack or one made from coconut.
Chocolate	Pure dark chocolate only, it is actually very good for you as it contains high levels of anti-oxidants and magnesium.
Hot chocolate drinks	Pure cacao, not cocoa, and mix with honey to sweeten.
Calcium	Dark, leafy green vegetables, carrots, almonds, figs.

Nutritional Lattes: The New "Coffee"

Some people feel they just can't live without their daily "hit" of coffee or caffeine, while others wish they could. We use it as an aid to better mental and physical functioning in our busy lives, but is it? Eliminating a stimulant like coffee from your diet may actually give you more natural energy in the long run, so let's find out why. Remember, if you are removing nerve system interference with chiropractic care, then you may not need the stimulant "hit".

There's also a myriad of other beverages that have flooded the market that can replace a café latte. They're pretty colourful, nutritious and delicious too.

One cup of coffee contains 50 to 100 milligrams of caffeine, which will produce a temporary increase in mental clarity and energy levels while simultaneously reducing drowsiness. Through its central nervous system (CNS) stimulation, caffeine increases brain activity, and also improves muscular-coordinated work activity such as typing. So far, so good. However, caffeine also stimulates the cardiovascular system, raising blood pressure and heartrate. It generally speeds up our body by increasing the basal metabolic rate (BMR), which burns more calories and stimulates appetite. Caffeine may initially lower blood sugar, but this can lead to increased hunger or cravings for sweets, and after adrenal stimulation the blood sugar rises again.

Caffeine also acts as a diuretic, meaning we lose excessive amounts of water by increased urination. By increasing respiratory rates, we lose more moisture through our breath, thereby adding to the cumulative dehydration effect. The cycle of stimulant effect followed by let-down as the blood levels drop may also contribute to emotional instability and mood swings.

It's evident that, as with most drugs, caffeine provides a short-term gain followed by a long-term loss which can be quite damaging to our health and wellbeing. So, is it easy to turn down that steamy latte or creamy cappuccino? No, it's not. Even with all we know now, habits and appetites and the desire for comfort are hard to resist.

Nevertheless, you can begin by reducing your intake and slowly replacing coffee with some delicious and healthy substitutes over time. The "coffee break" is great, but let's put the emphasis on "break" because you don't always need the extra stimulant, and there is no need to pass up a nice hot frothy drink with friends just because you've decided to take responsibility for your health.

In response to increased public demand for healthier options, the café society is churning out tasty caffeine alternatives with its chai lattes and dandelion coffees. It's extraordinary how many restaurants and chain coffee houses have jumped on the bandwagon. Some even call it an LSD – long soy dandelion – and it's listed as such on the menu.

The dandelion drinks taste remarkably like coffee, and the chai products contain aromatic Indian spices like cinnamon, cloves and nutmeg and taste wonderful with honey. You may have also seen the turmeric lattes, beetroot lattes, charcoal, matcha and many other varieties.

This way, you still get to meet for a social "coffee" with friends, have a warm drink to hold on cold days, break up your day with a refreshing treat, and apart from not stimulating or stressing your nerve system and dehydrating you, dandelion is actually great for digestion.

Parsley – Your Natural Breath Freshener

Pure Parsley Drops are found in some chemists and health food stores under names like "Pongoes", "Odour Go" and others. Parsley is an excellent natural way of eliminating bad breath due to such strong foods as garlic, onion, alcohol and many more.

While mints or breath fresheners work well temporarily, their action is limited to the mouth. Parsley works from the gut where the cause of the odour begins, and eliminates it within an hour of swallowing the concentrated parsley juice in the capsule. It is amazingly effective.

I like to cook with parsley a lot, especially by making a fresh GF tabouli salad which requires fresh flat leaf parsley as the base. You can even put it in a smoothie. I have a recipe for a kissable breath drink in my dating book #instalovers. Try it just once and you won't consider eating garlic without it again, and your clients, friends and partner will thank you.

A nickel will get you on the subway, but garlic will get you a seat.

Old New York Proverb

Limit Alcohol

Alcohol has been a part of human culture since the earliest written records, and for good reason. In moderation, it can aid digestion, act as a social lubricant, relieve stress, but in excess the health effects are disastrous.

Over time, excessive alcohol consumption creates yet another chemical toxicity and permanently damages the brain and central nervous system, as well as the liver, heart, kidneys and stomach. It's a simple statistical fact that heavy drinkers have shorter lives, and the life they have is much more prone to minor and major health problems.

Alcohol may accelerate normal ageing or cause premature ageing of the brain, and its effects can make some medical problems difficult to diagnose. For example, alcohol causes changes in the heart and blood vessels, and this can dull pain that might otherwise give warning of an incipient heart attack. It can also cause forgetfulness and mental confusion which resembles Alz-heimer's Disease.

By decreasing the amount of alcohol you consume, you will definitely turn back your biological clock. I am all about that! I don't drink much alcohol at all. If you decide to detoxify, begin by reducing the amount you drink in any one session, and slowly increase the periods of time when you don't consume alcohol at all. When celebrating or socialising, try to alternate alcohol with other drinks, so that you consume less. Try a sparkling mineral water with fresh lime, or a sexy cranberry juice. If you're a wine lover, you might like to explore the many organic varieties – they contain no preservatives and will be a healthier choice. There is also a distilled spirit that is non alcoholic that I found. It tastes incredible and it's without the ageing effects.

When is Alcohol Consumption an Alcohol Addiction?

Not everyone who drinks regularly has a drinking problem.

You might consider seeking help if you:

- drink to calm your nerves, forget your worries, or reduce depression
- gulp your drinks down quickly
- lie about or try to hide your drinking habits
- drink alone more often than with others
- need alcohol to help your moods
- lose interest in food
- feel irritable, resentful or unreasonable when you are not drinking
- hurt yourself, or someone else while drinking
- have medical, social or financial problems caused by alcohol.

Wonderful Water

It sounds incredible, but even though we are surrounded by water most people are dehydrated. There is a significant time delay between your body's organic water needs and your sensory awareness of it, so long before you have a dry mouth, or feel thirsty, you are actually suffering from dehydration.

The lack of water in your body will make you feel tired, disoriented and grumpy, and if the dehydration continues it can cause allergies, asthma and chronic pain. In the long-term, insufficient water promotes a variety of degenerative diseases such as heart disease and arthritis, as well as heartburn, weight and obesity problems, chronic constipation, headaches and migraines, child learning and attention disorders, depression and hypertension. If the *lack* of water does all this, what do you think proper hydration can do?

Why do adults need 2.5 litres of water a day? Because water *hydrates* your body, which has a host of beneficial effects – it improves energy and concentration levels, reduces the frequency of headaches and migraines, assists in weight loss, flushes the kidneys and helps prevent the formation of kidney stones, detoxifies the body by facilitating the removal of cellular waste products and reduces blemishes and plumps out wrinkles, giving your skin a glowing, supple, youthful appearance. Indeed, pure simple water is one of the best anti-ageing agents available, and by far the cheapest.

Until quite recently our society has not encouraged the drinking of water. It has promoted the consumption of soft drinks, kombucha, smoothies and shakes, tea, coffee, milk, fruit juice, alcohol – virtually anything but water, because there was no profit in it. However, times have changed, and water now means big money. Athletes carry and endorse glamourised bottles of expensive boutique water, celebrities are rarely seen unless clutching some imported variety to demonstrate their health-consciousness.

The world's sexiest and healthiest people are drinking so much water for very good reasons, and so should we. It seems we really don't appreciate something unless we pay for it, and now that water has become such a pricey status symbol, the truth about its great health-giving qualities is finally available to all.

Water; just because it's as accessible as the air, don't take it for granted – it is miraculous stuff.

Alkaline Ionised Water

Increasing your consumption of good quality tap or filtered water can transform your health, and play a big part in the healing of many degenerative diseases. However, there is another step to take when you're ready. Remember we touched briefly on how acidity adversely affects the human body? Well, water can be used to reduce it even further.

Alkaline ionised water has profound long-term effects because it alkalises your body, provides additional oxygen and is an effective new anti-oxidant. This is an additional source of oxygen provided in a body-friendly way, and the effect is similar to deep breathing, exercise, or sleeping in fresh air.

A water ionising unit can be installed at your kitchen sink or bench. It operates by filtering tap water, separating it into two parts by electrolysis – water containing acid minerals and water containing alkaline minerals. It then discards the harmful acidic portion and only allows the healthier alkaline water to flow out of the tap. It's actually easier to drink than normal water, as we can drink twice the amount of alkaline ionised water before feeling full or bloated.

As with most things, it's best to avoid extremes – you shouldn't drink alkaline water with a pH higher than 9.0, as excessive alkalinity can upset your body's biochemistry as much as excessive acidity. To make sure it's just right, I recommend a professional installation of ionised water at your home or office. Waters Co are my best recommendation.

Would You Like Water or Cola with Your Meal?

This may seem a somewhat trivial way to end a profound topic, but cola not only bears a large responsibility for unwanted weight gain and systemic acidity, it is also one of the many substances which may cause chemical interference to your nerve system.

- 75% of Americans are chronically dehydrated, and it is likely that the same percentage applies to half of the world's population.

- For 37% of Americans, the thirst mechanism is so weak that it is often mistaken for hunger.

The reason for these issues may well be the substantial cola intake of the developed and developing world.

Cola Facts

- The active ingredient in cola is phosphoric acid with a pH of 2.8 (highly acidic). It leaches calcium from bones and is a major contributor to the rising incidence of osteoporosis.

- It is extremely high in calories from refined sugar.

- Trucks carrying concentrated cola syrup must display the "Hazardous Materials" signs reserved for highly corrosive substances.

- In many U.S. states, highway patrol police officers carry two gallons of cola to remove blood from the road following car accidents.

Now we'll ask you again. Would you prefer a glass of water, or cola?

To maintain optimum health you need to drink 4–5 glasses of water a day. Some say up to 8 glasses is best. Take into account that during the colder months you may also be having herbal teas as a form of hydration or some may require more water because they're doing vigorous training, sweating, crying or anything where your body is releasing water.

Be connected to your body and its functions. Listen to what it needs.

Changes You Can Make

- Add more fresh, plant-based, unadulterated, whole grain, organic foods to your diet.

- Reduce your intake of packaged/processed foods, and cut out all MSG and microwaved foods.

- Make an appointment with a good nutritionist or naturopath for a complete check-up. When you begin a journey, it's helpful to know where you're starting from.

- Eliminate artificial sweeteners from your diet.

- Eat less deep-sea fish, and consider having your amalgam fillings replaced.

- Reduce your consumption of dairy foods.

- Replace iodised salt with magnesium or pink salts of the earth. These are rich in minerals as they have not been processed.

- Drink more pure water, and less alcohol and soft drinks.

Food is not just delicious, it's a source of life, and of healing as well. For the greater part of human history our only medicine was food itself, and the old saying "An apple a day keeps the doctor away" may contain far greater wisdom than we realised.

Remember, we should eat to live, not live to eat, and the most important and healthful change you can make to your diet is your own consciousness. We'll be discussing this vital component of life more in the last chapter, but in relation to food – simply be aware of your choices, and be grateful and appreciative when you eat. In fact, studies have measured this effect and found that although "junk food" should definitely be minimised in any healthy diet, the guilt that people feel when they eat it has a much more powerful suppressant effect on their immune system than the junk food itself. These facts are given to increase your knowledge, not your guilt, so don't be hard on yourself, just be aware. Mindful and conscious eating is all about connectedness.

5

Side Effects are Still Effects

*In Science, you learn "cause and effect",
not "cause, effect and side effect".
Side effects are still effects.*

Andi Lew

In the last chapter we saw how much of the food we eat comes at a price beyond the dollar cost – the unhealthy chemicals, both natural and manmade, that it contains. These hidden substances have unwelcome consequences when we consume them; they're called *side effects*, and they may be even more dangerous in the products we will be examining next – drugs, toxins, prescription medications and pharmaceutical-based beauty products.

If you already know and practice what we've covered so far, you likely take few if any medications because you live a wellness-based proactive lifestyle. But if, like most people, you've left your body's natural healing abilities unsupported by wise actions for too long, you're probably going to need "sick care". This usually involves some form of medication, artificial rather than natural, and side effects are an unavoidable sequel to taking any medication.

Every doctor has a large book in their medical library called a PDR, "The Physician's Desk Reference", and it describes the effects of every drug they are permitted to prescribe. The PDR contains all the drugs that have been found to be "safe for human consumption" and it lists not just the positive, beneficial effects, but also all the negative and harmful ones.

Did you know that there is not a single drug in that large volume without side effects?

We're going to reveal what some of those hidden effects are, so that you can be more informed about drugs, hormones and cosmetics that are commonly sold to the public.

Pharmaceuticals

Our modern world culture has become a chemical merry-go-round where we are given a drug for a specific effect (which we could often have achieved ourselves with a change in lifestyle), then given another drug to counteract the unpleasant side effects of the first drug, then yet another drug to help our body assimilate both of the first two ... and so on down the yellow brick road, forever chasing the elusive health that is our nature and birthright.

Many of the medications and hygiene products we use regularly contain toxic chemicals. You may not have noticed but the warm and comforting television commercials we see daily only give us half the story. They don't always mention side effects that come with their products.

Popular pain medications like paracetamol, aspirin and codeine are present-ed as perfectly harmless. It can be quite dangerous to take even common, over-the-counter painkillers on a regular basis. They're advertised as going straight to the localised source of pain but they're also bypassing the gut, affecting and going throughout the entire body too. And while the "family deodorant" is reducing body odour, what else is it doing that we aren't told? It's an irrefutable fact that all medications have side effects. In scientific terms, for every input there is a subsequent effect, and if you don't know all the effects, then you are not making an informed choice.

Effect

Something brought about by a cause or an agent; a result.

The power to produce an outcome or achieve a result; influence.

A scientific law, hypothesis, or phenomenon.

Side Effect

A peripheral or secondary effect, especially an undesirable secondary effect of a drug or therapy.

The dictionary definition suggests that effects and side effect are polar opposites; the effect is a desired outcome, while the side effect is an undesirable result of the same action. But whether you want it or not, the side effect is just as much a result of taking a drug as the effect. They are both effects, desired or not. Unfortunately, we can't selectively choose our effects – the side effect also occurs as surely as night follows day. When your doctor prescribes a powerful drug for you, are you fully informed about both the effects *and* the side effects? Do you mind the undesired effects less because they're labelled a "side" effect?

Science bases its research on the study of cause and effect, not cause, effect and side effect. Why is it, then, that all the negative outcomes are described as secondary *side* effects? Are they just the effects they don't want to draw attention to? Why are the negative effects written on medicine packets in such tiny print, and called "side" effect as though they were nothing to worry about? Isn't it almost a common joke about contracts to "watch out for the fine print"? You should be equally concerned about *all* the effects of any medication. The fact that you may not "feel" the side effect doesn't mean it didn't happen, or that you have less reason to be concerned about it. It's the fine print. As we've seen, symptoms are not a reliable measure of health.

As far as drugs and medications have come, there are still some frightening side effects that occur as the body adapts to the chemical changes or chemical interference and toxicity. Would you be surprised to learn that there is not one chemical found in medicinal drugs that your body doesn't already know how to produce? The vital difference is that the healing substances produced by the body are both natural and integrated, while the medical drugs are synthetic and disturbing. The more you learn about your body's innate power and intelligence to heal, the more you will trust it to take care of you when you take care of it.

Anything you take from outside the body is already produced in the body – if it's functioning correctly.

Ernie Landi, DC

So, all drugs produce side effects, whether short-term or long-term. If you take them, there *will* be various effects on your body. Side effects vary, so don't expect to necessarily notice them yourself.

They may be:

- undesirable and immediate
- time-delayed or cumulative, and occur later
- subtle, or non-symptomatic.

Antibiotics are an excellent example of a drug that has both beneficial "effects" and extremely undesirable "side effects". They are the most commonly prescribed medicine in the modern world, and their usage has increased so greatly over the past few decades that almost everyone has had a course of them. Antibiotics are useful because they destroy bacteria. However, there are good and bad bacteria, and antibiotics don't discriminate, they kill them all. The good bacteria are absolutely vital for our normal skin function, as well as digestive and immune processes, and we cannot live without them.

Apart from the dangers of over-prescription to humans, antibiotics are fed to livestock on a vast scale as a preventive measure against the unhealthy conditions that so many animals are kept in today. As we described earlier, through our own direct usage as well as the consumption of foods that have been fed antibiotics, we have created a culture of super-bugs – hyper-resistant bacteria that we can no longer safely treat with antibiotics.

The "effects" of antibiotics have been to kill off infective bacterial colonies, and the "side effects" have been the destruction of good, life-supporting bacteria. The most severe result has been the creation of deadly drug-resistant bad bacteria. Therefore, antibiotics have all three categories of side effects – some undesirable and immediate, some time-delayed and cumulative, and some subtle or non-symptomatic.

Another clear example is the common over-the-counter anti-inflammatory taken by almost everyone at some time, which includes products like aspirin and paracetamol (painkillers). Commonly used for pain relief, side effects are rare but they do happen. The lesser effects range from constipation to nausea and vomiting, while more severe side effects can be bleeding stomach ulcers and addiction.

The first three effects can occur more-or-less immediately, the ulcers take longer to develop and addiction is a subtle but ever-stronger effect, the result of long-term misuse of these drugs. While you may not feel them, the side effects will be taking place on a cellular level – as with any chemical; there is cause and then effect.

An Australian court judge has observed that a disproportionate number of the young criminals who appear before him were given Ritalin as children. Why were (and are) so many children being prescribed this drug without full knowledge of the possible repercussions? Perhaps the doctors themselves weren't aware of the side effects at the time, or there were simply no alternatives because the product was selling so well that research slowed, or the parents felt so desperate that they were willing to "try anything"?

Are you making desperate or fear-based choices? Are you researching and questioning everything? Take your time to understand all your options and find more than one opinion. No decision should ever be made through desperation. Allow it to come from inspiration. As new illnesses develop, we are still learning about the hidden side effects of drugs and medications once promoted by medical authorities as "safe", such as opium, morphine, lead, thalidomide, Celebrex and Ritalin. If you're not sure, the safest response is simply to say No to drugs – there *are* alternatives.

Side effects are not limited to drugs and medications; they are also in many of the unnatural or artificial products we use or consume in everyday life.

It may not be news to you that anti-perspirants and deodorants contain high levels of aluminium, but did you know that aluminium absorbed through the pores of your skin may be very harmful to your health? Side effects of using such seemingly innocuous products as aluminium-laced deodorant or anti-perspirant may be some of the most devastating illnesses of our time – Parkinson's Disease and cancer.

An increased risk of breast cancer may be caused by chemicals that mimic a woman's natural hormone – oestrogen. Aluminium-based compounds are being implicated more and more in this causation and products like anti-perspirants (which can have an aluminium content of 25% by volume). Aluminium has been shown to be able to penetrate through the skin and once inside the body, may cause significant health problems.

The Journal of Applied Toxicology published a review calling for further research to explore the increasing risk of breast cancer due to the use of aluminium-based products.

"Since oestrogen is known to be involved in the development and progression of human breast cancer, any components of the environment that have oestrogenic activity and which can enter the human breast could theoretically influence a woman's risk of breast cancer," says author of the review, Dr Philippa Darbre, who works in the School of Biological Sciences, at the University of Reading, UK.

Aluminium salts in anti-perspirants are a major source of exposure to aluminium in humans. It is often sprayed into armpits, inadvertently concentrating exposure near to the breast. In addition, it is often applied immediately after shaving, when the pores are opened and the skin is likely to be damaged and less able to keep the aluminium out. "It is reasonable to question whether this aluminium could then influence breast cancer," says Dr Darbre.

You may be concerned if you have been using these products for some time, but the best time to stop is now. Many people resist changing their type of deodorant for fear of becoming some kind of malodorous "health nut", but don't worry, we aren't smelly and we don't want you to be either.

After many years of testing nearly every alternative deodorant on the market, I know what works and what doesn't. So "hooray" for these solutions, and cheers to a slimmer chance of you ever developing Parkinson's Disease.

Firstly, understand the difference between an anti-perspirant and a deodorant. Think about the meaning of the words. A deodorant removes or masks odours, while an anti-perspirant actually prevents perspiration in the first place. As much as we may prefer not to perspire, it is a natural and vital bodily function, and we couldn't survive without it. Perspiration cools us and reduces excessively high body temperature, removes excess sodium from our system, and acts as a back-up toxin eliminator to our kidneys when they are overloaded or malfunctioning. Now that you have this information, it's easy to see why a deodorant is healthier than an anti-perspirant.

Remember how healthy expulsion is via an orifice? You release toxins through sweat, urine, excretions and our sneezes, coughs, eyes, ears, pores, and even our breath. Allowing for optimal expulsion is healthy.

Okay, we've eliminated anti-perspirants, but what *kind* of deodorant should you use? There are roll-on (non-aerosol) deodorants containing natural disinfectants such as tea tree oil which work well under the arms. Other pump spray and roll-on deodorants use natural fragrant aromatherapy oils. There are many effective varieties on the market, but you may need to re-apply during the day.

There is a vast number of crystal "deodorant stones" or roll-ons available at any health food store, and even the health food section of some supermarkets, but their effectiveness varies with the individual. Some users report total success and require nothing else to remain odour-free all day, while for others the results range from inconsistent to totally ineffective. It depends on your personal chemistry, so you won't know if they'll work for you until you try.

The best solution I've discovered so far is a crystal spray deodorant. After exhaustive and sometimes disastrous personal research, I find that with this product there is no odour. Try it and see if this one works for you. I do enjoy some of the other natural tea tree and lemon-scented roll-on deodorants, but you do have to re-apply them throughout the day.

Maintain hormonal balance, because armpit odour is in large part controlled by your hormones. That's why babies and children can sweat but still smell so sweet.

Men, keep underarm hair trimmed short. The longer it is, the more you will smell.

Finally, the simplest solutions are often the best, simply wash regularly.

I mentioned the possible connection between aluminium and cancer, but it is only one of many contributing factors. Understanding the effectiveness of medical treatment for this often-fatal disease may lead you to rethink how seriously you take the risk factors – if they can't fix it, then you don't want to "wait 'til it's broke". Prevention is the cure and it is really better to be safe than sorry.

Cancer Treatment – Effects and Effectiveness

This book is dedicated to the proactive approach to real wellness, and one of the greatest modern threats to your wellness is cancer. In fact, after iatrogenesis and heart disease, cancer is statistically most likely to be the cause of your death, so I want you to know more about it and how successful modern medicine has been in dealing with it.

At the turn of the 19th century, cancer was a relatively unknown affliction and certainly did not impact our families and society to the degree that it does today; that one in three people will have some type of cancer is extraordinary, and predictions are that it will rise to possibly one of every two. In the UK, it is estimated that by 2025 there will be at least another 100,000 cases of cancer if no other factors in society change.

Not only does research show that cancer is on the rise, but so is diabetes, heart disease, Alzheimer's, arthritis, chronic fatigue and many more diseases. With all our magical drugs and cures, why are the people taking them getting sicker? A great example of the growing problem that too many of us are having to face by ignoring the cumulative side effects of all our life choices is this increase of cancer.

In 1971, US President Richard Nixon announced a War on Cancer, and promised a cure by the 1977 bicentennial. In each year of the 25 years since, more Americans have died of cancer than the year before. The failure of chemotherapy to control cancer has become apparent even to the oncology (the study of tumours) establishment. The prestigious British medical journal *The Lancet*, decrying the failure of conventional therapy to stop the rise in breast cancer deaths, noted the discrepancy between public perception and reality. "If one were to believe all the media hype, the triumphalism of the [medical] profession in published research, and the almost weekly miracle breakthroughs trumpeted by the cancer charities, one might be surprised that women are dying at all from this cancer."

Noting that conventional therapies – chemotherapy, radiation and surgery – had been pushed to their limits with dismal results, the editorial called on researchers to "challenge dogma and redirect research efforts along more fruitful lines."

John Cairns, professor of microbiology at Harvard University, published a devastating critique in *Scientific American* in 1985. "Aside from certain rare cancers, it is not possible to detect any sudden changes in the death rates for any of the major cancers that could be credited to chemotherapy. Whether any of the common cancers can be cured by chemotherapy has yet to be established." In fact, according to Cairns, chemotherapy is curative in very few cancers, specifically testicular, Hodgkin's, choriocarcinoma, and childhood leukaemia. In most common solid tumours, such as those of the lung, colon and breast, chemotherapy is **not** curative.

An article titled "Chemotherapy: Snake-Oil Remedy?" appeared in the *Los Angeles Times* on September 1st, 1987. Dr Martin F. Shapiro explained that while "some oncologists inform their patients of the lack of evidence that treatments work … others may well be misled by scientific papers that express unwarranted optimism about chemotherapy. Still others respond to an economic incentive. Physicians can earn much more money running active chemotherapy practices than they can providing solace and relief ... to dying patients and their families."

Dr Shapiro is hardly alone. Alan C. Nixon, PhD, past president of the American Chemical Society wrote, "As a chemist trained to interpret data, it is incomprehensible to me that physicians can ignore the clear evidence that chemotherapy does much, much more harm than good."

In 1986, scientists from McGill Cancer Centre sent a questionnaire to 118 doctors who treated non-small-cell lung cancer. In their work, more than three-quarters of them recruited patients and carried out trials of toxic drugs for lung cancer. They were asked to imagine that they themselves had cancer, and then nominate which of six current trials they would choose. Sixty-four of the 79 respondents would not consent to be in a trial containing *cisplatin*, a common chemotherapy drug. Fifty-eight of them found *all* the trials unacceptable. Their reason? *The ineffectiveness of chemotherapy and its unacceptable degree of toxicity.* The survey concluded that if they were to contract cancer, oncologists would not use the chemotherapy they so readily provide to their unsuspecting patients.

This is all very alarming and confronting, but still somewhat theoretical to the majority of us who are cancer-free at the moment. But if you should one day be diagnosed with cancer yourself (and if you apply everything you learn here, that likelihood may be reduced), it can be difficult to know exactly what to do. Ultimately, only you can know the answer, if the time comes. Just make sure you do all the research, ask all the right questions, find a doctor you like, trust and respect, and look at *all* the options available before making your decision. Remember, it's *your* decision.

If you don't want to "wait 'til it's broke", then act now to increase your body's self-healing and self-regulating capacity with better nutrition, fewer drugs, chiropractic adjustments and all the other life changes recommended. They are safe, gentle, effective and have no side effects. In fact, given the right environment, your body's chemistry may be able to transform itself without you putting anything into or taking anything out of it, and without side effects!

It's good to know our excellent medical professionals are there in case of an emergency, but it's best not to put yourself in the position of having to rely on chemical solutions. It seems that almost every week another "wonder drug" is summarily pulled from shelves because of its dangerous effects revealed by more thorough testing. Were these effects or side effects? And are we valued customers or merely guinea pigs taking unwitting part in unannounced drug trials?

Vioxx was a powerful drug once prescribed to millions of arthritis sufferers, but when news bulletins around the world reported that it was linked to cardiovascular disease, including heart attacks and strokes, it was immediately removed from sale. Vioxx's negative impact was so great that disease almost appeared to be its major effect, with relief of arthritis pain merely a side effect. It is significant that we rarely hear about drugs with more side effects than actual effects, even though they obviously do exist. But it really doesn't matter what label a particular effect is given as we need to place more importance on all the effects before we decide to take any drug.

The reality is that every drug you take has an effect. That is the nature of a drug. That effect may range from outright cure to symptom relief, another symptom, a secondary illness or even death, so you want to be able to trust whatever you choose to put into your body. Remember, it's always a lot easier to put something in than it is to get it out. This is why the need for natural medicines has become so great in recent times, because even though these too need to be monitored, they are often free of the harsh repercussions of artificial chemicals.

So what should you do?

Care for yourself so that you don't get sick at all. I really can't remember the last time I was and if I was starting to feel out of balance, I would always ramp up chiropractic care, detox and all the lifestyle things needed and explained here. Prevention really is better than cure.

Try a natural solution first to see if your condition is amenable to natural-based care.

Boost your immune system so that your body will be strong enough to adapt to and/or resist whatever comes your way.

Do a little research on chiropractic and the immune system, and on immune-boosting products from fresh food sources and good quality nutritional products.

Former Merck CEO Henry Gadsden said in an interview with *Forbes* magazine that it was a shame he was not able to make Merck, one of the largest pharmaceutical companies in the world, more like the chewing-gum maker Wrigley's because then he would have been able to *"sell to everyone"*.

His views are interesting. What a brilliant business man.

So please, make sure that you ask questions to gain information and knowledge before making any decisions regarding your precious health. The answers may surprise and sometimes even shock you, but successful people are those who say and do the things that ordinary people don't. Your future is governed by your present, so choose wisely today.

Contraception

We've been exploring how to preserve and improve life, but there are also circumstances where many of us want to be able to prevent life from beginning at inappropriate times.

Contraception is a fraught topic for many, with strong ethical, philosophical and religious opinions on both sides. But in our culture, it comes down to a matter of personal choice, and choice cannot come without adequate information, which it seems is rarely provided.

This section on the drugs that alter hormones may make you think twice about your medication. If you are one of the thousands of women who have taken or are taking the contraceptive pill, it will be particularly valuable to you.

Men may think it has nothing to do with them, but contraception is a choice that both partners should be involved in. How medical contraception can adversely affect natural fertility and general health is something which is beneficial for everyone involved in the decision to understand.

Quit Messing with My Hormones!

What does the oral contraceptive pill actually do? It chemically alters your hormones to prevent pregnancy. This is the desired effect, but the side effects according to research from the National Cancer Institute, can range from weight fluctuation to moodiness, skin problems, cardiovascular disease and certain cancers.

For a fuller understanding of how the contraceptive pill works, and its side effects, let's look at the menstrual cycle. It is imperative for female fertility and conception, so without it there would be no human life on earth. Interfering with this amazing and complex intelligent body function with a contraceptive pill has serious long-term effects.

Menstruation begins in the sexually mature female body by a building up of the uterine lining (making it thick and plump) due to gradually increasing amounts of *oestrogen*, the hormone responsible for female maturity like breast development.

Follicles begin developing, and within a few days one or sometimes more matures into an *ovum* or *egg*. The ovary then releases the egg/s, which signals ovulation and an increase of luteinising hormone. The thickened and plump lining of the uterus is now ready to host and cushion an egg if it has been fertilised by a sperm.

The hormone *progesterone* rises at ovulation, and peaks shortly thereafter. If there is no fertilisation and no need for the lining to stay plump, the body's intelligence begins to slough off the lining of the uterus. The lining and blood supporting it pass out through the vagina, marked physically as the menstrual period, and the oestrogen levels go down. The average number of days between the beginning of each menstrual period is approximately 28 days (a lunar month), but this figure can vary significantly and still be considered as normal.

I've just described it in a somewhat clinical and chemical way, but what does it actually mean? Every "month" of its reproductive life, the female body prepares the uterus for pregnancy by first releasing oestrogen to thicken the lining for implantation, then creates an egg to be fertilised by a male sperm. If no fertilisation occurs, the body simply dismantles all its hard work to begin all over again next month, and all this incredibly complex creation and controlled destruction is accomplished through a finely balanced flow of hormones, without any conscious control by the woman. What an extraordinary example of intelligent self-healing and regulation.

What we find even more amazing is the part played by naturally created cancer cells in this process. *Cancer* cells? But aren't they dangerous, you may well ask? Not when a healthy body is producing its own in the proper amounts and conditions. We are actually made up of builder and destroyer cells, constantly renewing and replacing the different parts of our body all day, every day. Skin, stomach, eyes, heart, bone — all are made of cells and are built up and broken down at their own specific rates of growth and decay.

Incredibly, to accomplish this process the body produces cancer cells (vital destroying cells). Our immediate reaction to the very mention of cancer is usually fear and aversion, but astonishingly, all births are due in part to cancer. We fear it killing us, but actually we wouldn't be here without it. The cancer cells involved in conception are called *trophoblasts*. They are invasive, eroding and metastasising (cancer-like) cells of the placenta (the organ that connects mother to child and responsible for all nutrition and elimination). They are formed during the first stage of pregnancy, and the invasion of a specific type of trophoblast (*extravillous trophoblast*) into the uterus is a vital stage in the establishment of pregnancy.

Failure of the trophoblast to invade sufficiently may lead to miscarriage. The trophoblasts spread like cancer and eat away at the lining of the plump uterus to create a "hollow nest" for the fertilised egg to snuggle into. The intelligence in the body knows that the trophoblasts can be destructive, so as soon as the "nest" is created and their work done, they are quickly and efficiently destroyed by the body's own immune system. Trophoblasts become inert during pregnancy and are completely rejected by the foetus and mother at delivery – they are never incorporated into the bodies of either the mother or the foetus.

So now that we've examined the role hormones play in fertility, let's see what happens when we interfere with them through the oral contraceptive pill (OCP), hormone replacement therapy, excessive toxins or a poorly functioning nervous system. Approximately 39 million US women use some form of contraception, the birth control pill and the condom being the most widely used methods in the western world. Other methods include hormonal injections, implants, intrauterine devices (IUDs) and the birth control patch.

The oral contraceptive pill primarily prevents pregnancy by *preventing* ovulation. Another side-effect is the thickening of cervical mucus, which may prevent or slow sperm entry into the uterus. It also thins the endometrium (uterus lining).

This alters your hormones, changing your body chemistry to release excessive oestrogen and progesterone, thereby preventing it from releasing eggs. It's a clever and powerfully effective drug, using your body's own chemical messengers (hormones) against it. This obviously works against the body's innate intelligence, and confuses the cycle of the body being readied for implantation.

The OCP was introduced in the 1960s, became an immediate massive seller with no mention of anything but "negligible side effects" in the initial excitement, and continues to be so today. The women who took it then are largely the same ones taking hormone replacement therapy now.

It appears that a long-delayed side effect of taking oestrogen-dominant OCPs is a dangerously deficient generation of high-oestrogen, low-progesterone functioning females, who now must take high doses of progesterone tablets to neutralise the results of their years on this method of birth control. After years of artificially high supplementation, the body ends up forgetting how to produce these hormones on its own. It seems to be yet another "chasing our own tail" syndrome, and all the while women have been suffering the dangerous side effects of both types of medication.

I understand the importance of being able to choose the right time and place for conception, but contraceptive pills can have profound health effects. There are many other forms of contraception you can choose if you decide to stop taking the pill. I'd like to suggest you talk to your healthcare practitioner and family planning clinic before making a change. There is a wide variety of methods available, and they can help you find the method that is ideal for you – without side effects. Here are some examples:

Barrier Method

Barrier methods such as the condom and the diaphragm which physically prevent the sperm from entering the vagina to reach the egg. It can be a sensible option, but recommend the use of latex-free condoms where possible, which are less toxic and harmful to the highly absorptive vaginal lining.

Spermicide

This method involves a chemical that kills or disables sperm so that it cannot cause pregnancy. It comes in many different forms: foam, jelly, cream, film and vaginal suppositories.

Intrauterine Device (IUD)

This is a small, plastic, T-shaped stick with a string attached to the end. The IUD is placed inside the uterus and prevents sperm from entering by changing the lining of the uterus.

The IUD has been linked with health problems just like the menstrual cup, where the body may want to reject the foreign object. I had a friend who explained her uterus twisted, but luckily a chiropractor she was seeing picked up this and managed to do some internal palpations to untwist it, after she removed it. So, if these methods are considered, make sure you investigate it fully.

Natural Family Planning (NFP)

This method uses various techniques to determine a woman's exact times of fertility. By avoiding sexual intimacy at these times, or by using a back-up method during the window of fertility, pregnancy can be avoided. Techniques include the ovulation method and the symptothermal method (a combination of the ovulation method and monitoring of body temperature). There are also a myriad of period tracking apps and menstrual cycling health professionals that can help you with understanding your cycle and ovulation times. Dr Natalie Kringoudis at The Pagoda Tree is a doctor of Chinese Medicine, and hormones and fertility are her area of expertise.

The decision on which method to use is important, and can be overwhelming, so do seek personal advice from a competent and sympathetic professional. Most of us are not even aware of any options aside from condoms and the oral contraceptive pill. More than 16 million US women use birth control pills as their preferred method, and it is likely that a majority of these women "choose" birth control pills due to a lack of awareness of all the other suitable options available.

The list of side effects many women experience is as long as it is devastating, and of even more concern are the cellular changes which detrimentally affect the intelligent workings of the body as it strives to complete its normal and natural biological reproduction cycle. Oral contraceptive pills are not hormones like those produced in your body, they are artificially manufactured by pharmaceutical companies and contain synthetic hormones and preservatives.

Here are 4 important facts to know when considering your method of birth control, because if you have used these, they may have "messed with" your hormones.

1. Hormonal contraceptives are SYNTHETIC hormones.

The body is not designed to be exposed to these synthetic hormones, and especially in such high doses. Usage unavoidably increases the risk of developing serious chronic illness. It is up to you to decide if the benefits outweigh the tremendous risks. (See table of side effects on opposite page).

2. Birth control pills can deplete important nutrients.

Aside from the long list of potential side effects, birth control pills can deplete your body of vital nutrients. These nutrients include vitamin B2, vitamin B6, vitamin B12, folic acid, vitamin C, magnesium and zinc. Remember this from when we learned about assimilation of nutrition in the previous chapter? The "pill" is still medication and medication blocks micro-nutrition absorption, so keep this is in mind when you're trying to get to an ideal healthy weight or stay well in general.

Research on the pill (OCP) shows the following side effects:

- Live tumours

- Increased risk of heart attack and stroke

- Abdominal pain

- Migraines

- Blood clots

- Menstrual cramps

- Gall bladder disease

- Cramps

- Cycle irregularities

- Bloating

- Headaches

- Loss of sexual drive

- Trouble wearing contact lenses

- Nausea

- Irregular bleeding

- Increased risk of breast cancer, cervical cancer, endometrial cancer, ovarian cancer

- Fluid retention or raised blood pressure

- Breast tenderness

- High blood pressure

- Skin irritation or rashes at site of patch

- Mood changes

- Mental depression

- Miscarriages

- Vaginal infections

3. Depo-Provera hormone shots highlight complications.

A study in the May 2004 edition of the journal *Obstetrics and Gynecology* found that Depo-Provera users had declines in bone-mineral density averaging 3% each year. After two years, the losses in bone mineral density were approximately 6%, compared with a loss of only 2.6% among women using birth control pills.

In comparision, women using no hormonal contraceptives had, on average, a 2% increase in bone density during the same period. With the incidence of osteopenia (reduced bone density) reaching near-epidemic proportions, it makes no sense to expose young women to the possibility of further calcium loss coupled with toxins from our foods. With this attitude and approach to female health, negative repercussions may be inevitable.

4. There are much safer options than using hormonal contraceptives.

Barrier methods and NFP offer much safer, albeit less convenient, options than hormonal contraceptives. With NFP, there are no side effects and no toxic substances put into the body, and women often feel empowered as they, often for the first time, become aware of their fertility cycle. Understanding how your body works, and connecting to it is empowering. I do, however, recommend you learn the method from a reliable source, and if your fertility is particularly high you may want to use a back-up barrier method.

Dr Kringoudis is highly skilled in hormonal health and anything to do with fertility, menstrual cycles and women's health. Due to the high risks involved in long-term drug use, and because these other safer options exist, may I suggest to all the women who are reading this to stop hormonal contraceptives like the pill as soon as possible, but do it with the assistance of the experts.

So there you have the risks and side effects of most of the widely available and commonly recommended forms of birth control.

Side Effects of Chemicals in Everyday Items

Like most people, you may be completely unaware of the staggering quantities of chemicals in the items you use every day. We've been told that these products make our lives better, cleaner, and healthier, but the truth is very different.

Here are the obvious toxic chemicals which may affect your nervous system:

- Drugs
- Medications
- Alcohol
- Cigarettes

Less obvious toxicities that may affect your nervous system:

- Some household-cleaning products
- Beauty and personal hygiene products

- Mercury

- Adjuvants in some vaccinations

- Pesticides

- Additives

- Preservatives (found in most packaged foods)

- Environmental toxins

Using or consuming any of the above products might create side effects that may impair your health to varying degrees. Of course, some of them have both effects and side effects that we consider positive and beneficial, but like life itself, you can't get the upside without the downside tagging along. You already know the positive reasons why you use these products, so now consider all the negative reasons why *you should rethink it.*

Beauty Products

Like it or not, this is an age of health and beauty consciousness. Most of us would love to be younger, fitter, smoother, more beautiful, radiant and attractive, but we'd rather buy it than actually make it happen ourselves through a change in lifestyle.

People want to look and feel their best for as long as possible, as easily as possible, and therefore are willing to spend large amounts of money on cosmetics promising blemish removal, firmer skin, clearer eyes, fewer wrinkles or reduced weight. Too many of those promises are conditional, misleading ("reduces the *appearance* of wrinkles"), or empty and full of risks for the consumer.

Skin Care, Cosmetics and "Anti-ageing" Treatments

The skin is the largest *organ* in the body, made up of multiple layers of *epithelial tissues* that protect the underlying *muscles* and *organs*. The vain hope that surface creams can have any lasting effect is baseless, because your skin sheds and sweats constantly.

The nature of the industry dictates that cosmetic products are formulated for a shelf life of over three years, therefore most contain large amounts of preservatives to prevent spoilage. These preservatives are cellular toxins (poisons), otherwise they would be useless for their purpose – to kill bacteria and microbes. They penetrate the skin to a certain extent and many have been shown to cause allergic reactions and dermatitis.

Not all brands are with toxins though. During this wellness revolution, because of our self-education and research, we have asked for more natural brands. The more we demand, the greater the supply. Companies like Botani who has been developed by a naturopath, have our best interests in mind. They're safe, natural and nutritive.

Over 90% of all ingredients in commercially available cosmetic products though are of synthetic origin, and may carry all the associated health risks. And you can't tell if they're safe simply by looking – many chemicals used in cosmetics never cause visible signs of toxicity on the skin, but contain potent systemic toxins that are cumulative and can remain in the body for a very long time.

On the other hand, there is a wealth of information and practical knowledge available about genuinely natural products that have been used successfully for thousands of years. You may not always know about them, because the companies making them do not generate the vast profits needed to fund their multimillion-dollar advertising campaigns, but a little research will reward you far beyond the time invested. Furthermore, this is why I wanted to whet your skincare appetite with Botani, an Australian brand, to get you thinking about what you should be looking for and that it may not be what you see in huge advertising campaigns.

So let's find out about the side effects of some of the products (and chemicals) you probably *do* use, and perhaps you'll be more motivated to look into the alternatives. Below are only a few of the over 800 extremely or potentially toxic ingredients used in personal care products:

Propylene Glycol

Derived from petroleum products, this substance is commonly used in antifreeze, de-icers, latex paint and laundry detergent. It can cause irritation of nasal passages, and if ingested can cause nausea, vomiting and diarrhoea.

Research also shows that it alters cell membranes and can cause cardiac arrest. Commonly used as an additive to keep products moist, it is a cheaper, synthetic glycerine substitute.

Skin care products which contain this ingredient are often promoted as "helpful" to your skin, providing it with the moisture, firmness or vitality it is currently lacking. What you may not realise is that the condition of your skin may have been created by using cosmetic products with this or other equally harmful ingredients. Unaware of the cause, you choose a skincare treatment which contains the same irritating product that created the problem in the first place, thereby making it worse.

These chemicals, when absorbed into the skin, can alter its pH level, causing dryness and flaking. Hair and skin have a natural pH between 4.0 and 6.0 (slightly acidic). Synthetic cosmetic products will change the normal pH and can allow secondary infections to occur.

AHA

Alpha hydroxy acid is promoted as an anti-wrinkle agent, and is found in many skin and hair care products. Originally used as a cleaning compound and for tanning leather, it works by stripping the outer layer of the epidermis back to a "smooth finish" and causes the irritated skin to puff up and fill in the lines and wrinkles. Skin is exfoliated chemically instead of mechanically via abrasion, which dries and ages the skin. The FDA warns that strengths over 3% may thin the skin.

Acetamide MEA

Used in lipsticks and cream blushers to retain moisture, this ingredient causes adverse reactions and is toxic, carcinogenic and mutagenic.

Aluminium

Used as a colour additive in cosmetics (especially eye shadow) and in deodorants and anti-perspirants, aluminium has been listed as carcinogenic, toxic and mutagenic.

Benzene

This substance is a known bone-marrow poison, yet it is widely used in combination with other chemicals in many personal care products. It can cause adverse reactions and is carcinogenic, mutagenic and toxic.

Carbomers 934, 940, 941, 960, 961C

These are used as thickeners and stabilisers in creams, toothpastes, eye make-up and bathing products. They are known allergens that have a high acidic pH in 1% water solution. These synthetic emulsifiers can cause eye irritations and should be avoided.

DMDM

Otherwise known as hydantoin and used in the synthesis of lubricants and resins, this substance can cause dermatitis. Derived from methanol, it acts as a preservative, may release formaldehyde and is a suspected carcinogen. Rats develop cancer when injected with this chemical.

Elastin

Elastin is a protein in connective tissue. Promoted as improving the elasticity of the skin when applied externally, there is no proof for this claim.

Glycols (group)

This range of products is used as a humectant, which can be derived from animal or vegetable, natural or synthetic sources. In most cases it is used as a cheap glycerin substitute. Propylene glycol has caused liver abnormalities and kidney damage in laboratory animals. Diethylene glycol and carbitol are considered toxic. Ethylene glycol is a suspected bladder carcinogen. The FDA cautions manufacturers that glycols may cause adverse reactions in users. They have been shown to be carcinogenic, mutagenic and toxic.

Formaldehyde

Used in nail polishes and hardeners, soaps, cosmetics and hair growing products, it is often hidden under the name DMDM hydantoin or MDM hydantoin. Its trade name is formalin. The vapours of this colourless gas are extremely irritating to mucous membranes. It can potentially cause dermatitis, and ingestion can produce severe abdominal pain, internal bleeding, vertigo, loss of ability to urinate and coma. It is very toxic when inhaled, a severe skin irritant, and a suspected carcinogen. Its use in cosmetics is banned in Japan and Sweden.

Imidazolidinyl

This is the second most commonly used preservative in cosmetics. Colourless, tasteless and odourless, it is used in powders, baby shampoos, bath oils, colognes, eye shadows, blushers, hair tonics and lotions. It causes dermatitis, and if heated to higher temperatures this substance produces formaldehyde.

Lauramide DEA

Lauric acid is derived mostly from coconut oil and laurel oil. It is used as a base for soaps, detergents and laurel alcohol because of its foaming properties. Nitrosamines can form in all cosmetic ingredients containing amines and amino derivatives with nitrogen compounds, and nitrosamines are known carcinogens.

Parabens

This is a term used for petroleum-based butyl-ethyl-germa and propyl paraben, the most commonly used preservatives in a variety of personal care products, especially creams and lotions. It can cause dermatitis and allergic reactions.

Toluene

Obtained from petroleum; it is used as a solvent in cosmetics, especially nail polishes and dyes. It is also found in pharmaceuticals and gasoline as a blending agent. Resembling benzene, if ingested it can cause mild anaemia, liver damage, and may irritate the skin and respiratory tract.

Hair Care

Almost everyone uses hair shampoo on a daily or weekly basis, and complaints about irritations from shampoo are among the most frequently received by manufacturers.

Complaints range from scalp irritation to hair loss, eye irritation and severe hair damage. The vast majority of commercially available shampoos are loaded with chemicals that are hazardous to your skin and your health.

SLS

Scientific studies have proven that *sodium lauryl sulfate* or *sodium laureth sulfate* (SLS), found in most shampoos and conditioners, as well as toothpaste, skin creams and lotions, damages protein formation in the eyes. And to add insult to injury, after the damage has been done, SLS retards the healing process.

Kenneth Gree, PhD, DSc, Medical College of Georgia, warns that eyes affected by SLS take longer to heal. It can lead to cataract formation and eventually blindness, not only from direct eye contact but through long-term skin absorption. SLS can penetrate the eyes, brain, kidneys and liver, remaining in those organs for several years after use. It can also degenerate cell membranes, change the genetic information in cells (as it is a mutagen) and damage the immune system.

This chemical can also cause skin irritation, rashes, dermatitis, dandruff and allergic reactions. It contains ether and is toxic.

SLS, a hair care product, corrodes hair follicles, impedes hair growth and has been blamed for many cases of premature hair loss. Hair grows more slowly after exposure to SLS.

Studies have shown that SLS may enter the circulatory system with each shampoo or oral ingestion, and can react with other common ingredients of food supplements or cosmetics to form carcinogenic nitrates and dioxin. Exposure to SLS can lead to burning sensations, coughing, wheezing, laryngitis, shortness of breath, headache, nausea and vomiting, according to the Material Safety Data Sheet (MSDS) of the US government. A very high, hidden and unnecessary price to pay for clean hair, wouldn't you agree?

Alkylphenol Ethoxylates

Widely used in shampoo, it causes adverse reactions and research has shown it to be toxic, mutagenic and carcinogenic. It has been found to reduce sperm count, and to mimic estrogen in the body.

Ammonium Laureth Sulfate

Found in hair and bubble bath products, this substance contains ether and is easily absorbed by the skin. It is known to cause adverse reactions, and to be carcinogenic, mutagenic and toxic.

Coal Tar

Many kinds of shampoo designed to treat dandruff and flaky scalp contain this substance. It is disguised with names like FD, FDC or FD & C colour. Coal tar can cause potentially severe allergic reactions, asthma attacks, fatigue, nervousness, lack of concentration, headaches, nausea, and cancer.

Cocomidopropyl Betaine

This is used in shampoo in combination with other surfactants (substances which break up the surface tension of water to allow foaming). It is synthetic and can cause eyelid dermatitis.

Dioform

Many types of toothpaste and other tooth whiteners contain this substance. It has been known to damage the protective shell of tooth enamel by weakening it.

Fluoride

A toxic manufacturing by-product, this hazardous chemical was linked to cancer many years ago. It is supposed to arrest tooth decay, but scientists are now linking fluoride to dental deformity, arthritis, allergic reactions and Crohn's disease.

DEA

Diethanolamine is a synthetic solvent, detergent and humectant (emulsifier and moisturizer), widely used in brake fluid, industrial degreasers and anti-freeze. It is also found in hair dyes, lotions, creams, bubble baths, liquid dishwasher detergents and laundry soaps.

It can be harmful to the liver, kidneys and pancreas, and may cause cancer in various organs. Diethanolamine has also been known to irritate skin, eyes and mucous membranes, and poses especial health risks to infants and young children. Both hazardous and toxic, it forms nitrosamines which are known to be carcinogenic, and causes allergic reactions and contact dermatitis.

Dimethylamine

This is a secondary amine that can cause allergic dermatitis and is known to have carcinogenic properties.

Phenoxyethanol

This substance can be found under the names of arsol, dowanol EPH, phenyl cellosolve, phenoxethol, phenoxetol and phenonip. It has been known to cause severe allergic reactions.

Polysorbate-n (20–85)

Used as an emulsifier in cosmetic creams, lotions, cream deodorants, baby oil and suntan lotions, it causes contact sensitivity and irritation to the skin.

Polyquaternium

This substance can be carcinogenic, mutagenic, toxic and may cause adverse reactions like dermatitis and fatal drug allergies (anaphylactic shock). It may also cause increased sensitivity to muscle relaxants.

Sodium Oleth Sulfate

May contain dangerous levels of ethylene oxide and/or dioxane, which are both potent toxins.

Sodium (PCA/NAPCA)

Used as a conditioner for skin and hair, synthetic versions can seriously dry the skin and may cause allergic reactions. This styrene monomer can be carcinogenic, mutagenic, toxic, and may cause adverse reactions such as irritation to the eyes and mucous membranes.

Stearamidopropyl Tetrasodium EDTA

Nitrosamines can form in all cosmetic ingredients containing amines or amino derivatives with nitrogen compounds, such as this one. Nitrosamines are known carcinogens.

Talc

Derived in powder form from the mineral magnesium silicate, it can be hazardous to one's health and is toxic with prolonged inhalation. Some talc is found to contain amphibole particle distribution typical to asbestos, which is cancer-causing and a known lung irritant.

Triethanolamine (TEA)

Used as a pH adjuster and a coating agent for fruits and vegetables, it can cause severe facial dermatitis, irritation and sensitivity. Triethanolamine reacts with a specific acid to form oil in water emulsions, typically lotions, and may contain carcinogenic nitrosamines. Its main toxic effect in animals is due to its extreme alkalinity.

Now that you know more about them you wouldn't think of putting these toxic chemicals in your mouth, but you certainly don't want them on your skin either. Don't forget that skin is a *carrier*, not a barrier, so most of these chemicals are being absorbed through your pores and straight into your bloodstream.

What can you do to protect yourself and your family?

The best advice is to carefully read the labels on all products, and compare them against the list of harmful ingredients just given you. By choosing safer and more natural products, our purchasing power can change the way the cosmetic industry works. Remember, they are driven by economics rather than ethics, so if *we* don't buy it, then *they* won't make it.

And remember, it is already changing as we become more educated and demand more natural products. Even the commercial companies have now had to start changing the ingredients or at least the way they market to us, to meet our safe health demands.

By now you're probably beginning to see how many things you can do to advance your health and preserve your youth. No powerful drug can ever replace lifestyle choices, state of mind and personal responsibility in our quest for genuine vitality. Health is a living combination of *who* you are and *what* you do, and both are equally important.

The medical model (allopathic) looks at you as a collection of disconnected parts. If you have a sore stomach, you may be given medication to relieve the symptom without considering the effects of that medication on other parts of your body, or why your stomach was sore in the first place. The wellness model is all about connection, and the more we learn about our amazing body, the more we realise that no part is separate. It's all *connected*, and this approach is called "holism".

If you want optimal health, wellness, and youthful vitality, slowly incorporate everything you're learning here into your life, because it's really up to you. That's the *wellness* model.

As ye sow, so shall ye reap.

Galatians

Changes You Can Make to Get Connected

- Stop using anti-perspirants and aluminium-based deodorants. There are plenty of alternatives that can keep you sweet-smelling and healthy.

- Speak to your family planning clinic about the various methods of contraception. If you are currently taking the hormonal-based contraceptive pill, replace it as soon as possible with a safe alternative.

- Find out the side effects of whatever is prescribed for you. If you don't know all the effects of a drug or medication, then don't take it without more knowledge.

- READ LABELS. If you're going to put something in or on your body, then know what it is and exactly what it does.

Realise and recognise what medicine is best for – treating symptoms and disease, and emergency care. At times of crisis, it is truly wonderful. When survival is at stake, side effects are at best a secondary consideration, and in the emergency ward the emphasis is rightly on saving lives. Be grateful that drugs and surgery have come so far in modern medicine, but never lose sight of the fact that they are based on the philosophy of sick care, not wellness care.

Aim to swap your medications for the natural approach. Talk to your doctor so they can effectively co-manage with your other practitioner of choice. You may choose to work with a naturopath who will treat your symptoms naturally, and if your illness isn't too advanced you may get great results. You may elect to see a wellness chiropractor who will address the cause of your health challenge rather than just your symptom. Or you may choose to see both.

The next way to get "connected to wellness" is through the vital necessity of quality sleep for rejuvenation and regeneration.

References

Books

Aesoph, Dr Lauri ND, Your Natural Health Make over, Prentice Hall Direct.

Begoun, Paula, Don't Go To The Cosmetic Counter Without Me, 4th Edition, Beginning Press.

Hampton, Aubrey, Natural Organic Hair & Skin Care, Aubrey Organics.

Smeh, Niklaus J., Creating Your Own Cosmeceuticals-Naturally, Alliance Publishing Co.

Steinman, David & Epstein, Dr S., The Safe Shoppers Bible, John Wiley and sons.

Vance, Judy, Beauty to Die For, Promotion Publishing.

Winter, Ruth, The Consumer Directory of Cosmetic Ingredients, Random House USA.

Articles

Darbre PD. Metalloestrogens: An Emerging Class of Inorganic Xenoestrogens with Potential to Add to the Oestrogenic Burden of the Human Breast. Journal of Applied Toxicology 2006; DOI:10.1002/jat.1135.

Quinn, M., et al., Registrations of cancer diagnosed in 1994–1997, England & Wales in Health Statistics Quarterly 07 Autumn 2000. Office for National Statistics, p. 71–82.

Journals

Health News Newspaper, Triple R. Publishing Inc., Oregon USA.

Health Naturally Magazine, Feb/March 1997 page 2021, Zoltan Rona, MD, MSc.

The combined pill – Are there any risks? Family Planning Association (UK).

Cancer Research UK Statistical Information Team. stats.

team@cancer.org.uk.

Websites

www.ncbi.nlm.nih.gov/pubmed/9229520. Oral contraception and the risk of breast cancer. Plu-Bureau G, M Lé (1997).

6

HOW WELL ARE YOU RECHARGING?

The Slump of Sleep

Hippocrates realised that it wasn't the doctor who cured disease. Rather, an inborn force contained within a person's body was responsible for restoring health. To work in harmony with the inborn force and support nature's healing activities meant doing nothing that would infringe upon or disturb the natural process.

William J. Nelson

Sleep is underrated

Ah, sleep! We spend one-third of our lives in it, recover from the day's exertions every night, bond most deeply with our partner in bed, and receive some of our greatest dreams and visions in it. But for something that is so important, we give it remarkably little thought.

Over time, with the advancement of technology and the World Wide Web, we have become more reliant on connecting through technology or using technology to perform every little task. More screen time means less sleep time and you will soon learn why.

The very thing that helps us to get connected, also got us feeling disconnected. This in turn, has affected our sleep. How do we tune off tech?

What will help us become more connected? Rather than throw every advancement we have achieved out the window, we need to learn how to create balance, homeostasis in our body, and a balanced approach. Wellness is about balance in all areas, and the way we handle technology and sleep is no different. We just forgot about connection to ourselves and nature.

"A human being is a part of the whole called by us universe, a part limited in time and space. He experiences himself, his thoughts and feeling as something separated from the rest, a kind of optical delusion of his consciousness. Our task must be to free ourselves from this prison by widening our circle of compassion to embrace all living creatures and the whole of nature in its beauty."

Albert Einstein

How wonderful it is to be able to connect to all living creatures and the wholeness of nature itself. We have been able to connect and experience the love of a pet animal, the joy a baby brings to all, the wonder of magical lightning storms, sunsets and even the smell of rain as it leaves mother nature's clouds.

This divine universe we live in has so many gifts for us to share and experience. We know this because the wonders of a brilliant rainbow that appears in the sky for all to witness, can stop every human in his or her tracks, to observe its gift in what is the present moment. It's almost like a form of visual meditation that has been designed to enlighten and heighten senses.

The invention of the aircraft helped us to connect with other cultures, broaden families and experience new religions. The clever creation of a phone, then fax and now computer technology helped us to learn and see more.

We have now widened our circle and life experiences through connection to internet. Technology and social media are how we connect now. This is it. We are witnessing a cultural revolution. I have been able to meet new people and find like-minded groups and organisations As a result of our new-found social media, I am interested in social revolution. I have connected with the most amazing mentors and teachers, journalists, publicists, parents, entrepreneurs, and general community as a result of our technology.

But are we really connected?

Are we turning into the most anti-social society? Or can we use this social media social revolution to our advantage where we get to take what we need from it, give something back to be able to practice gratitude, yet still have balance?

And how do we stop to look within for the balance, if we are searching for ways to do so on the World Wide Web? You may even be reading this very "digital detox" book on a device as an audible or e-book. Isn't that ironic? Yet, it is okay. It's okay, because it just is. We are headed this way, so rather than swim away from the computer-era current, let's work with it to create a way to make it work for us.

I have been able to create the most wonderful connections with people within my immediate community as well as overseas as a result of our digital era. This though, should never replace or outbalance the connections and connectedness we need face to face, in the flesh and with nature.

As a certified food, lifestyle and wellness coach, my understanding of an overall holistic approach to life is where the ticket to personal freedom and wellness lies!

Being "well" is always a multi-factor approach. It really never is just one thing that you need to do. There's a multitude of things we need to do in order to create a more vitalistic lifestyle. The key is to start. Start somewhere. Because humans love progress. It doesn't matter what your personal end goal is because we are all unique, but if we are progressing, we are going to be happy. Once that ball gets rolling, guess what? You're going to feel more fulfilled, happier and will start to feel more connected!

And the term "wellness" is going to have different interpretations for each person.

What makes you well is going to be different to someone else's needs.

Our lives are so unique and so too will our diets and outlooks be, depending on lifestyle and even genealogy.

I started lecturing and inspiring others in their workplaces. Big companies such as Red Energy hired me to come in and help their staff get some more balance in their personal lives and whilst at the workplace. As a society, we spend up to 8 hours a day being sedentary in front of technology. Organisations are starting to realise the ramifications to our health and the importance of changing this. They may implement health professionals like me to advise and speak to employees, build a yoga room on site, or hire a massage therapist to come in once a week, or invest in buying staff gym memberships.

As a radio announcer, I saw new radio stations in Australia use the broadcasting area from a barstool-height desk too, allowing the announcer to stand should they wish to whilst on air. It's a fact that when we stand, and not slouch, our voice and energy levels can change.

I want you to start with just one thing to help enhance your sleep: a reconnection to yourself, your body and your community.

We are so connected to everything.

Let me prove it.

Did you know that women report that when they start to spend a lot of time together or to reside together, their menstrual cycles start to synchronise?

More beautiful synchronisation occurs and even more commonly than just synchnrosing with each other, is our synchronisation of the earth because women report to synchronise their menstrual cycle with the lunar cycle.

Lauren Geertsen, a nutritional therapies practitioner, discusses this very topic in her article published on her "Empowered Sustenance" blog.

> Random and uncomfortable periods are the effect of a diet and lifestyle that disconnects us from the rhythm of nature. Modern living means that most women abuse their bodies with various chemicals, antibiotics, prescription medications, the OCP (oral contraceptive pill), extreme emotional stress, the stress of over-exercising, refined foods, and more.
>
> Another key factor in hormonal imbalance is artificial light. It is widely known that the blue light from electronic device screens disrupts melatonin, wreaking havoc on our sleep cycles. Less well known is that our bodies are so sensitive to light patterns that women can manipulate other hormones by controlling the light at night. This is because our melatonin levels help control the hormones that regulate our periods, according to fertility specialist and author Kate Singer.

So, we have now learned we are that connected to the earth, the moon, and then sun, that when we try and even change that, our hormones become out of balance. Just wow! That's connection.

What about when birds fly in formation, or a school of fish are all swimming in unison? When one turns, do they turn to the others behind and yell, "Hey mate! In 200 m we will all turn left, okay?" No, they don't. They just do. They know. There's an innate intelligence and universal intelligence guiding us to all be the same.

Because we are connected.

What about other living creatures and things? Have you ever owned a pet dog and observed that they follow you around, and only decide to fall asleep when you do? And if you permit, usually at the foot of your bed.

What about babies? Did you know that our hearts, breathing and body temperature all synchronise when we co-sleep with our offspring? You only have to look at the works of professor and PhD sleep scientist James Mckenna, or read *The Science of Parenting* by Margot Sunderland to find out more about the mutual regulations of parent and child.

How we come into the world says a lot about who we are and the impact of our overall health, wellbeing and ability to heal or thrive. A disconnected birth because of drugs and intervention, may take some time to get connected again.

Leaving your baby to CIO (cry it out) or controlled crying methods can have huge psychological ramifications. I wrote about this very topic in my book *The Modern Day Mother: Babies and Sleep from Womb to One*. You see the human brain is in three parts when it is developing; the mammalian, reptilian and rational parts of the brain. They do not integrate and become one brain until about the age of five to seven years.

This means that when a baby is crying to be with you, the child literally feels like it is going to be eaten by a big lion, the rational part of the brain does not think the way an adult brain does until about age seven. The baby is acting in a primal state, the way the human body is designed to. Even though we have evolved as species and we live in safe houses, the way the human brain develops has not changed. The baby cries and releases too many stress hormones thinking it will be eaten by the lion and eventually gives up because it is too stressful. You might think you have taught your baby to "self settle", but they're actually feigning death, just like in the animal kingdom. It's a safety response. When you hold your baby close and allow it to synchronise heartbeats, breathing and body temperature, the benefits are mutual. It is a mutual regulation of heartbeats, breathing and body temperature and when mothers breastfeed lying down with their baby under their arm in a C shape, and both 'mum and bub' fall asleep in this position; they release a hormone called CCK which stands for cholecystokinin, which puts them both into a deep sleep. A twenty minute nap will feel like two hours! This is the best way for new mothers and babies to get quality sleep.

Sometimes, those unsettling cries to be held might actually be a hormonally connected plea for you to settle down, breathe and sleep too. What if we learned to trust our babies and our instincts? It can be a little annoying in the modern world, when we have jobs and other responsibilities

The bottom line is, all living creatures are connected, and we are designed to be connected to other life. This helps our wellbeing. This is why doctors have suggested us humans get a cat or dog for companionship to help with depression sufferers. When we are connected to other lifeforms, because we are designed to love this way, we are more well.

Yet, we live in a big city most of the time, and in big houses, far away from each other and we pretend that we have it all going on and don't need anyone's help. But we all suffer at some point, needing connectedness. We used to live in communities, close to each other and caring for one another. We took it in turns to cook, clean and look after children. We hunted together, gathered together and built villages together.

So now, we try to create connectedness and have been successful in doing so through practices like yoga, meditation, mindfulness and prayer. When we worked together with nature, that was our yoga and meditation, or connectedness, because we connected with each other **and** the earth at the same time.

However, when we are not present or in the now through any of the above, we become disconnected.

Here are perfect examples of just how connected we are, even to the planet itself!

- Did you know, the percentage of water within our bodies is about 70–80%?

- So too is that percentage in the earth itself. Yes, the earth is about 70–80% water!

- What is really astounding is that so too are plants! Yes, plants are also made of 70–80% water.

All life forms are just that, life.

When we nourish our bodies with more plants, we are not only hydrating, but giving us more life. And we then also acknowledge our connection to the earth and environment. Some call this mindfulness or mindful eating.

Want more stories about connection? Well, how connected is this?

We all need movement. The earth and us, needs movement to survive. Movement runs the brain. All living things have a nerve system. So we all need movement. As a qualified chiropractic assistant having run a wellness chiropractic centre for 13 years, I saw all too well the damaging effects and ramifications of not enough movement in our sedentary lifestyles.

My son asked me one day, "Mum why does it need to be so windy for?"

I explained that one of the reasons was to stir and shake things up. Movement is life. For example, the wind moves the water and creates negative ion effects and moves the trees to shake off dead leaves or drop seeds so more plant life can grow.

When water is still, that water starts to become murky, dull, flat and well, you get the drift (pun intended), lifeless!

We too, need movement to create more life. If we don't move, we die too. For example, in my studies as a chiropractic assistant, I understand that the nervous system, which is our brain, spinal cord and nerves that branch off of that, need clear communication. Misalignment, or vertebral subluxation, creates an interference to the nerve system.

We need proper movement, nutrition, less toxicity and even less emotional stressors, to minimise it all.

Furthermore, as cliched as it sounds, "if we really don't move it, we will lose it". That's why when us humans land in a hospital from an accident, we need a physical therapist to come and help us move our limbs to keep movement. You see, movement runs your brain. Use movement and chiropractic care to reconnect mind to body.

When we take a painkiller-type medication for a headache, we are disconnecting brain to body. We are switching off pain signals. This might be crucial in emergency, after trauma or during an operation, but for overall health and wellness, chiropractic allows us to have clearer communication from brain to body and may even create a heightened consciousness.

So here are 6 **connectors**:

1. Become more compassionate.

2. Feel general wellness.

3. Create a higher consciousness.

4. Connect with your community.

5. Find your soul's purpose.

6. When you turn off tech, consciously go inward or into nature.

To achieve the above, yes, you are going to need to do the below big three words: TURN OFF TECH.

Have you become addicted? With any addiction, we fear the unknown of what may happen when we remove the addiction from our lives. The phone is a great example. We all know the feeling of FOMO ("Fear of Missing Out") when we turn it off. We are addicted to the immediacy of the contact. So what if we weren't missing out, but instead are gaining, by turning off tech?

Let's make a list of the possible gains, besides the abovementioned:

- Better sleep quality
- Better clarity
- Improved relationships
- General feelings of wellness

What if we thought a little more left-field?

- The possibility of meeting someone authentically in the flesh by looking around you
- Improving communication
- Less car accidents
- Saving battery power

So there's so much to gain. I am sure you made a few lists in your head too after being inspired by reading some of the possible gains above.

The good news is I am not going to make you go cold turkey, or even give it up forever!

Jokes aside, after returning from a trip to America where I toured my 5th book *Real Fit Food* in October 2015 was when I realised that we, as a society, have become more disconnected with a situation that was supposed to connect us. Using technology may have brought us together in some ways, but it also brought us further away from our actual selves. The problem is often the solution. You may seek solace in this very notion, when things don't always go the way we plan. Maybe they're guiding us to lessons for growth?

I didn't find this new digital age sad. I think it's genius! Well, actually - it's both.

If it weren't for apps and social media, I would not have been able to make the many connections I have made over the recent years. I wouldn't have been able to find last-minute hotels and accommodations at really affordable rates. And I have met some incredible people, companies and watched some of the most genius of ideas through video blogs and searching.

At what cost though?

The reality is that it does affect and have an immediate effect on our sleep.

Let's talk about the **slump of sleep**.

Have you realised your sleep isn't as good or as long as it used to be? It's not just about the fact that we are reading emails, texts and searching online shopping catalogues or dating apps for more hours now. It's not just about the extra time spent. It's about the time of day we are choosing to spend it.

We need to at least carefully choose the time of day in which we use our technology for the sake of sleep. I suggest considering even at least a chosen number of days or indeed nights when you choose to not look at your computer screens or phones right before you go to sleep.

I think some people find it really hard to stop something they love. What if I told you that you can still have wellness and better health, just by at least choosing to stop an unhealthy habit only for a period of time, particularly at night.

There's no need for this "all or nothing" attitude. Just "sometimes" is okay, and that is balance.

I will highlight the importance of why we must try to at least sometimes do this switching off. Don't just take it from me. Look at what one of my clients, who is a surgeon, has to say about how technology disturbs our sleep.

We return home when sun is setting and the reduction of the sunlight allows the pineal gland to secrete melatonin which makes us feel sleepy. It is the nature's way of telling us that it is time to go to bed and get rest.

Unfortunately, the pervasive glow of electronic devices at nighttime is disrupting our circadian cycle. The lights from the electronic devices such as computer screens, smartphones and tablets often stay on throughout the night. These devices emit light of all colours but it is the blue spectrum light that suppresses our melatonin production and tricks our brain and body that it is daytime. As a result, we are systematically sleep-deprived because of how society works against our natural clocks. Studies has shown that sleep deprivation increases the risk of mood disorders such as depression and anxiety and reduces our ability to cope with stress.

Our modern society also encourages children to stare at the electronic device screen all night. The danger with disturbing children's sleep can affect their brain development. Sleep is important for learning, memory, brain development and health. We're systematically sleep-depriving kids when their brains are still developing, and we couldn't design a worse system for learning.

Many epidemiology studies also demonstrated that shift workers have higher incidence of cancers (e.g. breast, colon, prostate). It has been suggested that the disruption of our body's biological clock weaken the immune system. Previous animal studies showed that disruption of the biological clock can lead to accelerated neurodegeneration, loss of motor function and premature death.

This is an important issue that people don't talk about because our society is so addicted to 24/7 lifestyle, profit-driven society that bombard us with more electronic gadgets which will result in unintended consequence in the human evolution.

Dr Benjamin Wei
MBBS, PhD, FRACS

So let's invest in the word "**balance**" word right now. We are getting the sleepy picture when it comes to how it impacts our overall health nightly.

You see, when it comes to our diet, lifestyle, health and the way we connect now, we can have it all if we just implement balance. Balance is key.

So if you are going to use TURN OFF TECH as one of your "things" you incorporate into your daily plan and 5-day digital detox, then may I suggest you choose to turn it off at least an hour before retiring?

Alternatively, you may choose to not look at devices at all for 3 nights a week. The rest of the week, you can look at it all you want, especially if you have a night job that requires you to do so. Just make a plan to turn it off at night a bit before bed, or have a number of days where you do not look at it at all at night. Go for it the rest of the time! At least your body will have those quality days/nights to adapt.

Just do something else before you go to sleep, anything at all, to allow your eyes and brain to start to produce the hormones they need to allow you to have more quality sleep. When your hormones are happier, your body will work better, and you will in turn be happier as a result of being more well.

That blue light that is emitted from your screens robs your brain of the hormone melatonin that helps you to go into a sleep. You can take melatonin supplements, or wear blue light blocking glasses which help with 50% of the light emissions, but remember that supplements are meant to supplement. They're only meant to be there for a short period to get you back on track. Our bodies make all the right drugs the we give it the right environment.

What about the other environmental factors that create a slump of sleep?

Most mattresses have an effective lifespan of less than 10 years, the cheaper ones considerably less, and yet the average couple hangs on to their old mattress for more than 17 years! Only 11% of people replace their bed because it has become uncomfortable. Isn't it incredible that *89%* of us are prepared to spend 25 or 30 *years* in an uncomfortable bed? It's time to consider whether your bed may be contributing to your health problems.

The 2002 National Sleep Foundation (NSF) poll found that 74% of adults experience some sleeping problem a few nights a week or more, 39% get less than seven hours of sleep each weeknight, and more than one in three (37%) are so sleepy during the day that it interferes with their normal activities. A significant amount of this deprivation can be traced to improper mattresses, but once you have bought a new bed or mattress you can rest assured that, according to a French study, you are likely to fall asleep more quickly, wake up less in the night and gain up to an hour more sleep per night.

So how do you tell if your mattress needs replacing?

If the mattress sags in the middle or is just plain lumpy, it has to go. If it's too narrow, too short, too hard, too soft, or simply too smelly, then out with it.

If you and your partner find yourselves rolling together whether you intend to or not, that's another sign your bed has had enough. You may be one of the 16% whose partner cuddles them all night long, but your bed, not your personal magnetism, could be the reason.

Sleep deprivation is a serious issue, as it can be a major contributing factor to poor health, and the cause may be traced through your bed and pillow to your spine itself.

One benefit of being asleep is that our senses no longer need to be on high alert, monitoring every stimulus in the environment and alerting the brain to changes and possible dangers. In order to facilitate "turn-off" mode, our awareness of our surroundings needs to be different so that we can maximise relaxation and rejuvenation. We darken the room and close our eyes to minimise visual stimulation; our world goes quiet and the ears turn off to all but loud or unusual sounds; our skin stays sensitive to temperature changes but our responses stay below the conscious threshold, which is why we don't always awaken when it's too hot or cold with the blankets either on the floor or still wrapped snugly around us. The purpose of all this sensory shutdown is to allow us, and particularly our brain, to *rest* long and deeply.

How does that relate to your spine? Well, this general shutdown does not apply to specialised nerves called "proprioceptors". They provide constant feedback to the spine from the joints because we need to be aware of gravity all the time, so that we know where we are in space. That's why our simian ancestors didn't fall out of the trees, and why we don't fall out of bed. It's thanks to our joint receptors that we can perform the surprising feat of sleeping in unfamiliar and sometimes very narrow beds, move about quite vigorously all night without waking, but always stay within the confines of our mattress.

Thus joint, muscle and ligament receptors around the spine are always active, and if your mattress is too hard or too soft or too lumpy to allow your spine to relax naturally, then the receptors receive too much stimulation. Poor spinal function or spinal nerve irritation (subluxation) may feed nociceptive (negative messages or pain) input to the brain. If pain is feeding into the nervous system, then it can't shut down and it becomes very difficult to rest as the brain is constantly receiving negative signals from the body.

You may not be aware of this constant low-level negative (nociceptive) stimulus, but your brain and body are, and they suffer for it. You can treat the pain with drugs, but they bring adverse long-term effects – it's always wiser to go to the cause rather than the symptom.

By removing nerve system subluxation and allowing your brain to receive positive signals, it switches "off" as it rejuvenates.

Negative messages can also disturb the part of the brain that controls alertness and consciousness. Each night we follow a path that takes us from normal waking consciousness down through the different stages of sleep; every one of these stages is important for complete rest of the body and mind and all are more likely to be experienced with undisturbed sleep. This path follows a predictable pattern of REM (rapid-eye movement) and NREM (non-rapid eye movement) sleep throughout a typical 8-hour period. Each of these states alternates every 90 minutes.

NREM: 75% of the Night

As we begin to fall asleep, we enter **NREM**, which is composed of Stages 1–4.

Stage 1 – Light sleep; midway between normal consciousness and entering sleep.

Stage 2 – Onset of true sleep; disengaging with the environment, breathing and heartrate are regular, body temperature drops.

Stages 3 and 4 – Deepest and most restorative sleep; blood pressure drops, respiration slows, energy regained, hormones released for growth and development.

REM: 25% of the Night

This stage first occurs about 90 minutes after falling asleep and increases over the later part of night. The body becomes relaxed and immobile, the muscles shut down, the brain is active and dreams occur as eyes dart back and forth, breathing and heartrate may become irregular. It is important for daytime performance, and may contribute to memory consolidation.

Spinal problems can prevent us from reaching all these phases in REM and NREM sleep. That's why one of the common reports I hear after a chiropractic adjustment is, "I was tired, went to bed and fell asleep almost as soon as my head hit the pillow, and had a wonderful night's sleep". The effects of chiropractic on sleep are real, and chiropractic care is essential to restore normality of signals from the spine that map out body positioning in space while we sleep.

If you have subluxation, then chiropractic adjustments can correct it, removing the consciousness-altering pain signals and restoring normal proprioceptive joint input to the brain. If the spine is under any joint stress, a pain-free night of deep sleep is unlikely and many people may develop insomnia due to undiagnosed spinal problems.

Sleep is our time for healing, and the cumulative effect of poor sleeping patterns is a serious concern.

Newborns and infants need a lot of sleep in several periods throughout a 24-hour time period because they're laying down new neural pathways and growing new tissue. Adults function well on one uninterrupted sleep period of about eight hours, if it is *quality* sleep. Our sleep patterns may change as we age, but the importance of good sleep for better health remains the same throughout life.

Having a warm shower or bath before bed will warm the inner core and allow for better melatonin production. Try to wash and bathe right before you sleep and do not turn on tech after this. Out of the bathroom and into the bedroom! Wear a shower cap so that you have dry hair and can make that lovely transition from bath to bed, quickly!

A healthy bedroom environment is going to have no technology or EMFs in it.

Remove all technology from your place of sleep. This includes unplugging them from the wall. Turn off all devices and the wi-fi connections.

You may also want to look into ways to harmonise the effects of the electromagnetic radiation.

Plants, certain types of crystals and EMF harmonisers can help to negate the electricity and dirty electricity, but the radiation is a whole other ball game. This is why finding out where the wi-fi is weak is crucial to have time and space where you are disconnected from technology and connected to nature.

Barrister Ray Broomhall has been educating his clients on how to understand manmade EMR, learn steps for litigation if you are electromagnetic hypersensitive, and access potential remedies. He helps you identify the sources of non-ionising EM radiation like a mobile phone communications tower that might be near your place of dwelling or work, SMART meter, wi-fi router, and other devices.

You can also measure the emissions to ascertain safety levels and obtain a medical opinion as to whether or not the EMR emissions or proposed emissions are or could pose a risk of harm to your health. If risk of harm to health is advised, then one can request that the medical practitioner advise on recommendations as to what needs to be done to remedy the situation. Examples of recommendations might be that you are not be exposed to EMR emissions from the tower or device, or use a cable instead of wi-fi. You may wish to provide your medical practitioner with a link to the Bio-initiative Report 2012 (updated 2017) "A Rationale for Biologically-based Public Exposure Standards for Electromagnetic Fields (ELF and RF)" which can be downloaded at https://bioinitiative.org/

In Australia, you can find your mobile communications tower on the RFNSA website at https://www.rfnsa.com.au. Enter your suburb in the search field, identify the tower, click on it and retrieve the EMR report and compliance certificate to find the emissions or proposed emissions in your area.

You can find telecommunication licences for emitters using HAPS and satellites on the Australian Communication and Broadcasting Commission's website.

You can also ask your doctor to refer you to a specialist medical practitioner who consults EMR patients on a regular basis or, even better, one who has appeared in either a court or tribunal on EMR issues. Your lawyer may also be able to refer you to a medical specialist if needed.

Contact a building biologist to conduct a report as to the level of EMR emissions in your home, then obtains quotes for shielding purposes, such as shielding mesh, clothing, shielding paint to shield not only your person but also your house (inclusive of land). A building biologist should be able assist in this regard.

Removing EMFs, EMR and/or providing potential ways of removing the effects or the input can have a profound impact on your sleep, and overall health.

Tips for Good Sleep

- Avoid alcohol, as it can lead to disrupted sleep.

- Avoid stimulants such as caffeine (coffee, tea, soft drinks, chocolate) and nicotine (cigarettes and other tobacco products) close to bedtime.

- Exercise regularly, but complete your workout at least 3 hours before bedtime.

- Establish a regular relaxing, not stimulating, bedtime routine (e.g. taking a bath or reading a book before turning off the light)

- Create a sleep-conducive environment that is dark, quiet, comfortable and preferably cool. Remove EMFs and EMR where necessary.

- Spend more time in nature getting earthed and connected to our planet.

How's Your Sleep?

Do you:

- snore loudly?

- know (or have been told) that you stop breathing or gasp for breath during sleep?

- feel sleepy or doze off while watching television, reading, driving or engaged in daily activities?

- have difficulty sleeping 3 nights a week or more (e.g. take too long to fall asleep, wake frequently during the night, wake too early and cannot get back to sleep, or wake unrefreshed)?

- feel unpleasant, tingling, creeping feelings or nervous-ness in your legs when trying to sleep?

- have heart palpitations, night sweats and brain buzzing like tinnitus?

- have interrupted sleep (e.g. nighttime heartburn, over-sensitivity to light or noise, temperature fluctuations, bad dreams, discomfort or pain)?

You may be having nerve system interference, hormonal issues or EHS. You will need to make some lifestyle, health and environmental changes as discussed earlier.

Additionally, the proper mattress, pillow and chiropractic care may alleviate or even remove some or all of these symptoms of improper sleeping alignment and support.

What to Look for in a Bed

Since everyone is unique and all are at different stages of healing their subluxations, everyone's mattress will be slightly different. It's a good idea to consult with your chiropractor to find the bed that's exactly right for you, and you can also look at the range of beds that are endorsed by the Chiropractor's Association.

If you are buying a bed with a sleeping partner, try the bed out together for several minutes to get a good sense of how it feels to both of you. A new bed can be a significant financial investment and is vital to your health, so take your time. Don't be shy, talk to the salesperson while you're lying down. If you are buying online, you might want to check the return policy.

Foam mattresses have become popular with advances in foam technology – they are better for asthma and hay fever sufferers, but possibly not for the chemical-sensitive. The best, which can be quite costly, are made of heat-sensitive memory foam which moulds perfectly to your shape. Cheap foams tend to break down quickly and are not a good investment.

With the more substantial mattresses, you'll find that a pocket spring design will last longer. These are more comfortable and are ideal when two partners are of different weights. Comfort and price are dictated by the number of pocket springs, as well as the padding that may sit as a memory foam on top of the mattress for extra comfort.

A healthy bed should be quite firm, because if it's too soft you will find it sagging under your weight, which can distort the spine. And never put a new mattress on an old base, as the condition of the base is just as important as the condition of your new expensive mattress, and can have just as big an impact on your good night's sleep.

Remember that as the mattress ages, you're going be changing as well (hopefully for the better with regular chiropractic care) and will therefore require different support. A good bed is money well spent, and some quality manufacturers offer a guarantee to exchange your mattress for another when it's time for an upgrade.

Pillow Talk

Your pillow is as important as your mattress for a good night's sleep, and regular replacement is necessary. The sole purpose of your pillow is to support your neck in the ideal position, a lordotic curve (the banana bend).

Here's a simple test to check the state of your lordotic curve. Stand naturally erect with your heels and shoulder blades against the wall, and see if the back of your head touches the wall. If the answer is No, then this means your structure needs some help from a chiropractor, and you need a better pillow too. The further your head is away from the wall, the more correction you need.

If your pillow is too thick, your head will be pushed forward too much. This puts a strain on your delicate neck joints and contributes to the loss of the banana curve in your neck. If you feel more comfortable sleeping on a big pillow or two pillows, or a pillow that is too flat, then it may mean you've already lost that natural curve and have a series of subluxations in your neck. The old pillows need to be replaced, but don't just throw them away. Place them under your knees when lying on your back, which can take the weight off your lower spine and allow for more comfort.

Sleeping on your stomach is the worst position of all, because the neck is twisted round unnaturally with kilos of pressure from your body weight. A pillow tailored to your needs and measured by your chiropractor can make sleeping on your stomach impossible, which will break the habit and be much healthier for you in the long run.

People with neck problems need a shaped foam pillow which is thicker at the neck section and provides the best support, and those without neck problems would be well-advised to consult their chiropractor to make sure they don't develop any. Buy from a reputable supplier, or better still from your local chiropractor, to make sure that you get the right size and shape for your individual neck. I recommend TPI pillows and you will see their information at the back of the book.

7

PERCEPTION IS EVERYTHING!

The mind is its own place,
and in itself can make a heaven of hell,
a hell of heaven.

John Milton
Paradise Lost

Well, we've been working pretty hard so far, so let's take a moment to have a little fun. You've earned it, and we learn more when we are having fun!

Follow the instructions above these images, and afterwards we'll discuss why.

Read aloud the words inside the triangle below.

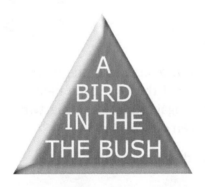

More than likely you said, "A bird in the bush," and if so, then you failed to notice that the word THE is repeated twice! You may not believe it, so look again.

Next, let's play with some words. What do you see here?

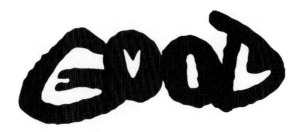

In black you can read the word "GOOD", but in white is the word "EVIL" (inside each black letter is a white one). This is not just perceptual, it's also philosophical and visualises the concept that good cannot exist without evil (or that the absence/opposite of good is evil).

Now, what do you see?

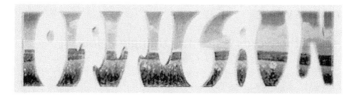

You may not see it at first, but the white spaces create the word "OPTICAL", and the landscape behind reveals the word "ILLUSION". Look again, and you'll see two reasons why this painting is called an optical illusion.

And again, what do you see here?

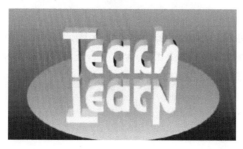

This one is quite tricky. The word "TEACH" reflects its complementary opposite "LEARN".

And finally, what do you see here?

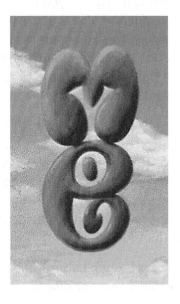

You probably read the word "ME" in brown, but when you look through ME what's revealed is "YOU"! Do you need to look again?

Surprising, amusing, and interesting, but why give so much attention to illusions? Because they reveal a profound truth, not just about the limitations of perception, but about reality itself. We've learned that when it comes to health, you can't always trust your senses. The body is so adaptive and resilient that not all illnesses reveal themselves through symptoms, and when they finally do, sometimes the disease is so entrenched that it's too late to do anything about it.

You've just had an undeniable experience of how fallible your senses and perceptions can be, even in something as simple as an optical illusion. Just as you may not have perceived what's right in front of you, your sense of your own health may also be an illusion.

Whatever you saw in the pictures above, you were probably quite certain that you were right – you could see it, so it must be true. But what happened was that by selectively focusing on one side of an image, the other side was hidden from you. Only when you saw both sides did the whole picture come into focus, and not until then were you able to appreciate not just the two sides but also the intelligence that created them.

We may perceive only one side of a truth yet firmly believe we have the whole picture. Until we personally experience something it remains purely theoretical, so that's why we took the time to "play" with these images – to communicate in an undeniable way that sometimes what we and almost everyone else believes and knows to be true may actually be only half the truth, which is therefore an illusion of the full picture.

We have been trained by our culture and our own physical reactions to believe that illness and disease somehow contradict this universal principle of wholeness, and have only a negative side that should be gotten rid of as soon as possible. We have looked at illness or symptoms and seen only the inconvenient or painful negative aspects, so we haven't understood them for what they really are – a healing response by the intelligent body to an unbalanced situation, and a message to us about what changes we need to make in our lives to optimise our health, vitality and overall quality of life, both in body and in mind.

There are none so blind as those who have eyes but will not see.

Unknown

Perception?

We're talking about perception, but what exactly *is* it? It's not about *what something is* as it is about what we *tell ourselves* it is. To the farmer, rain is a welcome gift to be celebrated, to the wedding planner or picnicker it's a curse – it's the same rain, but with two very different reactions. So it's clearly not about the rain itself but rather the perception of it, based on value systems. We guide our lives based upon our *perceptions*, perceptions are all about *information*, and the *quality* of our information is based on two factors:

- Our value system, derived from our social culture and family upbringing.

- The quality of the messages that our brain receives through its various receptors; that is, visual, auditory, kinaesthetic (touch), olfactory (scent) and gustatory (taste).

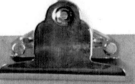

True Story

One morning, I opened my closet and was surprised by the number of green clothes hanging there.

I realised that over the last five years they'd been slowly accumulating, and when I looked around I noticed that my house was also full of green things – furniture, cushions, paintings, cloth, art objects ... they were everywhere. What made it interesting was that I suddenly remembered how I used to loathe green. It had been the colour of my high school uniform and brought back many negative memories, so I avoided it whenever possible, and now my whole life was filled this colour.

> I began to think more about it, and realised that the colour itself hadn't changed, but my perception of it had undergone a complete transformation.
>
> It was a small thing, but it stimulated me to look further and I began to wonder how many people had sparked either misplaced trust or unwarranted aversion because their appearance, accent, clothing, or job unconsciously reminded me of people in my past I had positive or negative associations with. How often had I been too open and given too much, or been too closed and given too little, without even knowing why?
>
> I realised that my unexamined perceptions were not always reliable, even though they "felt right" at the time, and I resolved to try and see people for who they really were, not who I thought they were, because I now knew that everything had two sides – like the colour green.

Let's face it – the only true science is Quantum Physics. There is an equal and opposite energy to everything.

Ignorance means to see only one side of things, to "ignore" the other side that makes up the whole picture.

How many people, places, things, and events in your life have you closed your heart and mind to, not because of who or what they were, but because of whom or what you thought they were? How many beliefs and attitudes have you unquestioningly accepted because you trusted the authority? They weren't necessarily malicious, they may have truly believed in what they said, but that doesn't make them right. Don't forget that wisdom is much less common than knowledge, and nobody, no matter how educated or powerful, has all the answers in this amazingly complex experience called life.

'It's what you learn after you know it all that counts.'

John Wooden

Perceptions are ultimately neurological. We've just discussed how to improve the *quality* of the information you take in, but what about what happens to that data inside you? You have neurological receptors all over your body in addition to your five senses that take in information from the environment and transmit it to your brain through a complicated series of electrochemical interactions. When they reach your brain, those signals are interpreted and become thoughts. But what if your nerve system is subluxated and not functioning properly, distorting or losing messages altogether? Your perceptions would also be distorted or inaccurate, and you could find yourself doing and saying and believing things that are in direct opposition to the best interests of your body and mind, *and feel absolutely correct in doing so.*

It's a little disturbing, isn't it? So what I am asking you to do is to stop taking accepted beliefs (society's or your own) for granted and begin to truly think for yourself.

The Two Sides of Science

Science has been an unquestionable gift to humanity. Without it we'd still be living in mud huts with a life expectancy of around 30 years, so all praise and thanks where it is due. But like everything that exists, science also has two sides, and its achievements have blinded us to the effects of that hidden side.

There is a branch of so-called scientific research that is actually "propaganda science". This type of science is not governed by objective testing, but is quite masterful at partial truths, selective data, statistical manipulation, and the skilful presentation of only one side of any issue it is used to promote.

Technology has created the gift of worldwide instantaneous communication, but the downside lies in the controlled selection of the information that constantly bombards us. We have become not only the most informed generation in history, but also the most conditioned, programmed beings the world has ever known. Our thoughts and beliefs are carefully shaped and moulded, and they are often not our own. So whose are they, and where do they come from?

An elderly lady came into my wellness centre one day. She was very distressed, almost too fearful to leave her house, and actually felt the world was about to end. It was clear she'd come to us more for company than healing, so we sat her down with a cup of tea and talked a while. It turned out that her husband had died some months before, and she'd spent the entire time since then sitting at home alone watching the news. That selective reportage had become her reality as stories of crime, war, destruction and murder filled her home and her mind. Those things definitely do exist, so her perception of the world was not untrue, but it was extremely *unbalanced*. The world does have honesty, kindness, peace and beauty, but because those images don't sell as well, she was given an overdose of the other side and felt the world was a terrible place.

Just a little warmth and attention did a lot to calm her down and remind her that television is not all of life, but she had been genuinely frightened by the unbalanced vision of the world she'd been given. The old saying *"You are what you eat"* is partly true, but you're also what you see and read and hear and think. We are all *influenced* by our environment, but we don't have to be *products* of it. It would be wise to give attention to what surrounds you on a daily basis.

Just like that elderly lady, we've all been implanted with thoughts and ideas by a flood of media input every day, and it creates needs and fears in us that may not be real.

Just like the pandemic experienced in 2020, we too saw a lot of sadness, destruction, death and illness, but I refuse to believe there wasn't a silver lining, if not many. It's quantum physics, remember? It had to be there, but we must exercise our minds to look for it. We must choose to see the gifts, the lessons and the connectedness it brings too.

Where does all this one-sided belief system come from? Hold onto your chair for some background on the dissemination of information in our modern world. Once you understand the origins of the current system of media control, you may be more inclined to question what it tells you.

The "art" of modern public influence began in the early part of the last century, with the work of Edward L. Bernays, known and revered in advertising circles as the "Father of Spin". He adapted many of the principles of psychology created by his famous uncle Sigmund Freud, and applied them to not just interpreting but controlling human behaviour.

Bernays personally created the science of advertising, mass persuasion, and "spin", which means the ability to reinterpret something to mean whatever you choose. With his extraordinary chronicle *Propaganda*, he dominated the public relations industry until the 1940s, and his legacy continues to afflict us to this very day. If you'd like to know more about the man who has had such an unwelcome effect on your life, an excellent source is *Trust Us, We're Experts*, by Stauber and Rampton.

Here are two far-reaching examples of Bernays's work to influence public opinion:

- **Sell World War 1 to the American public**
  This was one of Bernays's first assignments. The U.S. government wanted to enter the war, while the great majority of Americans felt it was a European conflict and wanted nothing to do with it. Bernays worked with the

Committee on Public Education and successfully sold the First World War to the American public with the slogan "Make the World Safe for Democracy". (Ewen)

- **Sell cigarettes to women**

  A few years after his successful war campaign, Bernays was hired to popularise the idea of women smoking cigarettes, which had previously been limited almost solely to men. The 1929 New York City Easter Parade was the product of Bernays' organisation, and it featured the "Torches of Liberty Brigade" in which suffragettes marched while smoking cigarettes as a mark of women's liberation. The ensuing publicity from that one event made it socially acceptable and *politically responsible* for women to take up a habit that has since been responsible for or contributed to the deaths of literally millions of their descendants.

It was Bernays who later came up with the advertising angle where the tobacco industry used endorsement by the AMA (American Medical Association) to prove that cigarettes are beneficial to health, which lasted for nearly 50 years. You can still find those amazing (in light of present knowledge) tobacco ads in old issues of *Life*, *Time*, and *Post* magazines from the 40s and 50s, and they illustrate how insidious and effective his work was on an unsophisticated, uninformed public.

Bernays described the public as "a herd that needed to be led" and that this herd mentality made people "susceptible to leadership", and he became the best at providing that "leadership" by putting his employers' products or concepts in a desirable light. This rationale served a purpose in its time, as Stauber describes it; "This is a logical result of the way in which our democratic society is organised. Vast numbers of human beings must cooperate in this manner if they are to live together as a smoothly functioning society. In almost every act of our lives, whether in the sphere of politics or business, in our social conduct or our ethical thinking, we are dominated by the relatively small number of persons who understand the mental processes and social patterns of the masses. It is they who pull the wires that control the public mind."

However, the selling of ideas is not a secret to those who make a living from it. Companies such as Philip Morris, Chlorox and Pfizer have supported this type of marketing. But the best PR goes unnoticed by the general public. In the past and present, that list includes vaccines, pharmaceutical drugs, chlorine, household cleaning products, global warming, leaded petrol, genetically modified foods, aspartame, forests and lumber, dental amalgams, alternative medicine, cancer research and treatment, air/land/ocean pollution, war, and the images of politicians and celebrities.

Bernays was very clever, and developed back-up plans to support his work whenever his (mis)information was questioned. People may not trust an advertising agency, but they are much more likely to be receptive to the findings of an independent research institute with a name like the Global Climate Coalition when it produces a scientific report stating categorically that global warming is a fiction. With a policy inspired by his particular genius, he set up "more institutes and foundations than Rockefeller and Carnegie combined." (Stauber p 45) He would quietly support the industries whose products were being evaluated through his "independent" research agencies which would churn out "scientific" studies and press information to support whatever position he was paid to sell. The tactic worked, and these "research" companies were and still are given official and trust-inspiring titles such as:

- Temperature Research Foundation

- Manhattan Institute

- International Food Information Council

- Center for Produce Quality

- Consumer Alert
- Tobacco Institute Research Council
- The Advancement of Sound Science Coalition
- Cato Institute
- Air Hygiene Foundation
- American Council on Science and Health
- Industrial Health Federation
- Alliance For Better Foods
- International Food Information Council
- Global Climate Coalition

And who are you to question the power and wisdom of such legitimate-sounding and prestigious companies? Bernays then went a step further and provided press releases announcing research "breakthroughs" to every radio station and newspaper in the country, thus saving overworked and time-poor journalists the trouble of doing their own research. They could just copy and paste the findings he created for them, and as a result the news was literally written by corporate PR firms. All of these practices continue today, albeit in more sophisticated and subtle forms.

There are a number of things that we have been told so often, in so many ways, that we forgot to consider where the idea really came from and just how true it is. Consider the following:

- Pharmaceuticals restore health.
- Vaccinations are the 'only way' and always bring immunity safely.
- The cure for cancer is just around the corner (every week).

- When a child has a fever, always give paracetamol.

- Hospitals are always perfectly safe.

These are stories we take for granted because it's just "common wisdom" but in actual fact those statements have been created through the investment of billions of dollars.

There is some truth in there somewhere, but let's look at how we accept them unquestioningly. How often have you thought to question any of the listed assumptions? Certainly by reading this book you've already started to question a few. Now it's time for you to determine how you feel and think with the additional information presented here.

Change of Perception #1: A Symptom is Not Your Enemy, but Your Friend

As we've already seen, symptoms like vomiting, purging, fever or excessive sweating are the body's intelligent means of dealing with a health challenge. The power that created your body and runs it through the medium of your nerve system causes you to demonstrate these functions (a.k.a. symptoms) and expel the toxicity. These are the actions of the power that is healing your body, although it may not feel like it at the time. It's not how you feel but how you feel about or perceive that feeling which determines your healing and wellness.

Once you understand this, your perception of these bodily functions will change dramatically. The old perception has dictated that we should suppress these healthy reactions and the two most common ways of doing so have been drugs and surgery. The new perception is to nurture and encourage the body to express its symptoms in order to reach a new and improved state of function, after it has learnt to deal with the stresses.

We care for people in our practice who, although they have not yet been diagnosed with a disease and show no physical symptoms, are unhappy in their life, work and family, feel under constant stress, and are merely enduring life rather than living it to the fullest. Allopathic medicine would say these people are healthy and require no treatment, but that's not how they would describe themselves. So that brings up a big question: who is actually healthy?

If we associate health with an absence of symptoms and sickness, how do we explain a vigorous woman who has no symptoms one morning, but whose mammogram that same afternoon reveals a cancerous lesion? She looked and felt fine, but it was an illusion created by the reliance on symptoms to determine healthcare.

But rather than thinking about illness as an indication of our mortality, consider if this symptom is there to help you discover how to live.

Those who focus on the negative perception of symptoms may find that if they do present with an illness, that fact alone may become the centre of their existence, taking over their life and defining their state of wellness. Rather than them having a disease, the disease has *them*.

Others carry on as if they are well (which according to our definition they are) and do all the things we've discussed that support living a wellness lifestyle, but change their priorities so that their focus becomes on living life rather than fighting disease. Your perception of your body's expression of sickness and health will determine what kind of person you are, and how you meet this challenge if and when it comes.

It may be the lack of understanding of the true nature of wellness that leads to disease, which raises the fear that something is wrong, which in turn represses the immune system and exacerbates the disease, and this cycle of misunderstanding creates the downward spiral that we look to drugs or surgery to rescue us from.

Understanding and trusting your body, making healthier choices, and adopting a wellness strategy designed to better adapt to stress – all of these impact the disease state far more profoundly than conventional reactions.

Change of Perception #2: Vomiting May be a Sign of Health

You are actually very healthy if your body is able to eliminate toxins through its portals. Contrary to popular belief, the time to be concerned is when you *can't* manifest symptoms through these systems.

We know it isn't a pleasant image to visualise but vomiting or expelling toxins is one of the healthiest things you can do. Remember that your body is on your side.

It is designed to self-heal and self-regulate. As long as we don't interfere with it the body works just fine. But if we introduce toxins by drinking too much alcohol, overeating, or eating bad food, the body will try to protect you from the negative effects of these.

Your body's quickest way of expelling a toxin is through the mouth, but vomiting is an unpleasant experience, and if we don't understand its role in our health, we will call it bad and try to avoid doing it. This has led to a wide variety of drugs on the market that suppress this normal reflex. But remember that vomiting is a response to toxicity, so if you repress it the toxin stays inside you.

If you repress the vomiting reflex, your body's next level of response is to send it out the other end. If you take something else to stop the diarrhoea, then that can weaken your immune system so that you become vulnerable to colds and flu. Your intelligent (and patient) body then dutifully tries to sneeze or cough the germs out into the air, but if you don't understand why it does that you may take a medication to stop *that* process. The next escape route for the chemical or bacterial toxins is the pores of your skin, which can result in pimples, rashes or eczema. The more severe the toxicity the more extreme the eruptions, so the medical response to such an affliction is a cortisone cream which clears up the condition by pushing the toxin back into the body that is so desperately trying to get rid of it.

Eventually the body gives up trying to expel what it knows doesn't belong in there and tries to encapsulate or isolate the toxins in various parts of your anatomy. Years later, when you are diagnosed with a major health challenge and the doctor says that the tumour took at least a decade to develop, you think to yourself, *But when did all this start? How could this happen to me?* Well, now you know.

You can see that every step on this path of ill-health was a reaction to a misunderstood symptom, a perception of what would make us well. This pattern will be repeated until there is a revolution in our understanding and treatment of symptoms and disease. You can't arrive at truth when you begin with false premises, it's like trying to reach a destination with the wrong map – you won't get there unless you throw it away and seek new guidance. So in the quest for health and vitality and longevity, here is your new map:

Disease is nothing but your body's way of ridding itself of whatever compromises your health!

So, the next time you cough or vomit, instead of automatically reaching for a pharmaceutical suppressor, ask yourself and your primary healthcare practitioner if what you are experiencing may be a detoxification or elimination process. Of course, you must monitor this with your primary healthcare practitioner, but your *perception* of sickness and health can change from one of aggrieved resentment to an appreciation for a hard-working and intelligent friend, and that can make a lifetime of difference.

To take in a new idea you must destroy the old, let go of old opinions to observe and conceive new thoughts. To learn is but to change your opinion.

B.J. Palmer, DC, PhC

Change of Perception #3: There are No Negative Events, Just Negative Perceptions

There was once a girl whose parents divorced when she was very young. She was extremely upset because she loved her father, but he was no longer a part of her life and there was nothing she could do about it. As a result, family became her highest value, so when she eventually had children of her own it gave her great joy.

Then her own marriage ended, and she was devastated. With her dreams of a happy family dashed and feeling like a failure, she also lost her job and suddenly there she was – approaching middle age, with children to support, no husband, no job, no money and living on charity. As a result of this overwhelming series of misfortunes she became deeply clinically depressed.

She had nowhere to turn to and nothing to do, so one night she sat down at her computer and began to write a story to cheer herself up, or at least distract herself from her misery. Into that story she poured all of her pain and loss and hopelessness, all her hopes for love and friendship and wealth and a true family. To her surprise, the story took over and sometimes she simply couldn't type fast enough to keep up with the flow of words that came from "somewhere else". As the manuscript grew, her depression lifted, almost as if by magic – she just didn't have time to be depressed when the story called to her with such urgency to be born. When it was finished, she sent it off to a publisher and waited for the rejection notice she was sure would come by return post, but she didn't really care because the writing itself had begun to heal a wound inside her.

That young woman was J.K. Rowling, and almost everyone on earth knows what happened next. She went on to become the most successful (and wealthiest) author in history, whose books and the films made from them have brought joy and wonder to millions of children and adults around the world.

She has said since that she wrote them to give Harry Potter a family, because it was what she herself most longed for. Everything in those books came from the apparent "tragedies" that beset her; poverty, two lost families, feeling alone and helpless, deep depression, and powerful forces seeming to seek her destruction. She healed them by writing about wonderful banquets and friends and games, having a great purpose in life, discovering hidden powers within, and finding love in unexpected places. Even her depression added to the power of the books when she personified it as the "dementors", horrifying creatures which sucked all joy and light and life from their victims, and gave Harry the power to overcome them.

Looking at her early life from only one side, it would be hard to see it as anything but a painful tragedy. But when we know what her challenges led to, the story becomes one of triumph and courage, and all the sorrows are revealed as hidden gifts that eventually transformed her life and touched the world. So were those experiences bad, or good, or possibly … both? When we look with only one eye at anything, we are (half) blind. Only those who look with both eyes, at both sides, can see truly.

Experience is not what happens to you, it's what you do with what happens to you.

Aldous Huxley

By now, many of your old belief systems may have begun to change as a result of the things we've covered so far. One of those beliefs may be your idea of what wellness really is. Did you believe that health and wellness were about being happy all the time, without pain or symptoms?

But realistically, we all know, in hindsight, that "negative" times can also be blessings; that's when we may find out who our true friends are, we learn to look inside more deeply and find resources we never knew we had. It's a time when the barriers can come down and we finally open our hearts to loved ones or to turn to a higher power, when real character and strength are born.

Ian Thorpe, Olympic swimming champion and multiple world-record holder, was asthmatic and allergic to chlorine. Oprah Winfrey, billionaire and the most powerful woman in the world's entertainment industry, was born into extreme poverty and abuse in the deep south, but turned her experiences into a drive to champion the rights of women and children around the world. Albert Einstein, Nobel Prize winner and a man who has become synonymous with the word "genius", did not speak a word until he was three years old, was terrible at arithmetic, and the headmaster once called his father in to tell him that young Albert was a dullard who would never amount to anything.

They all began with huge handicaps, what the world would call bad and negative things, but what was different about them was their *attitude*. They all turned their stumbling blocks into stepping stones, and became world leaders not in spite of but *because* of their "handicaps". Every coin has two sides, and they're all made of precious metal, you just have to know how to look at them.

There's an old saying, *"Pain is God's megaphone"*. It's a way of getting your attention when you haven't listened to the earlier, gentler messages. Pain is in your life for a reason, and if you perceive it wisely, you'll use it to make healthy changes in how you live.

We've all tried to avoid sadness, but constant manic happiness is not a healthy way to live either. In life the two always come together in alternating cycles, and the more extreme the elation, the more intense the subsequent depression.

Those who seek constant *"happiness"* are setting themselves up for sadness, if only because they can't ever entirely escape the other side, because life *is* the ups and the downs. The key to true health is to recognise the balance, making those ups and downs less extreme.

Remember that there is nothing stable in human affairs; therefore avoid undue elation in prosperity and undue depression in adversity.

Socrates

Did your doctor forget to explain that having a healthy perspective is fundamental to your health? The WHO says that optimal health is not just physical, it's about emotional wellbeing too. When it comes to optimal health, emotional wellness is vital, and *perception* is the key to both.

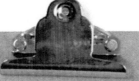

True Story

In my 20s, I experienced my first "broken heart". The boy and I worked together so I quit my job. So there I was, not only heartbroken but unemployed and with a severe case of sciatica that riddled me with pain. I couldn't think clearly, and was feeling so depressed and helpless from my reactions to all these "negative" events that I went to see a doctor, insisting that she give me anti-depressants for my misery. She refused. Instead, she took the time to ask why I thought I was depressed. When I told her of my broken heart and all the other challenges, she listened patiently, then explained that I was going through a natural reaction, that it was normal to feel depressed after such events, and that I was in fact depressed but not in a depression. I will never forget her wise and kind words: "Now, I can give you anti-depressant medication, but it will change who you are, and who you are is good."

That wonderful woman gave me permission to feel, to go through a grieving process for my lost love, and then helped me address the causes of my feeling depressed. I felt supported and had new hope for the future. I firmly believe that doctor helped save my life.

What's interesting is that she didn't change my circumstances at all, she just changed my attitude toward them, and that changed everything.

Who looks outside, dreams; who looks inside, wakes.

C.G. Jung

Have you ever heard the saying, *"I gave up happiness, it made me too sad"*? It's a thought-provoking phrase which reveals that it's our quest for happiness that is turning us into a Prozac nation. At what point did we lose sight of the fact that life was about both happiness and sadness in proper measure?

But having said all that, it's still a fact that pain hurts, illness is at the very least challenging, and we would prefer to minimise our experience of that form of wellness. You'll never get rid of them, but there are two strategies you can adopt that will reduce their impact on your life:

1. You can master your reactions when they inevitably arise, not giving in to fear or doubt, but respecting your body's intelligent ability to take care of itself and aligning yourself with it.

2. You can adopt a proactive life style that will maximise your body's ability to deal with whatever happens, reducing major disruptions to your life.

We've already discussed many ways to do both of these things, so now let's look at a few more simple ways you can bring a bit of joy into life, particularly if you are experiencing a challenging or difficult time.

- Get a pet, or take a neighbour's dog for a walk.

- Surround yourself with vibrant colour and pure white.

- Open your windows to let the natural air and light in.

- Fill your home with plants and breathe them in or eat them!

- Light candles and be present, pray or meditate.

- Take a short afternoon nap daily. It reduces stress, and your cells can rejuvenate while you rest.

- Reduce your stress. Unmanageable stress in your life creates acidic conditions in your body, which can lead to and exacerbate illness.

We are spending billions of dollars in this country fighting disease, and precious little on discovering ways to regain and maintain health – chiropractic is just that.

Tedd Koren, DC

Change of Perception #4: Drugs are Not Designed to Boost Your Immune System

Your immune system plays an enormous role in the overall health of every cell and tissue in the body. Not only does it protect us from everyday challenges like colds and flu, it also repairs damaged joints, helps fight against cancer, and slows down the ageing process.

Chiropractic prefers to build up your resilience and resistance to illness and disease, rather than trying to change the environment to suit a weakened body. Because the nerve system controls the immune system, and chiropractic is about removing nerve system interference, chances are that if you are having regular chiropractic treatment and your diet is good (or even organic), you probably experience less sickness. And when you do become ill it passes much more quickly. You really can't control what happens to you mentally or physically, but you can definitely influence how your mind and body *react* to what happens to you – and that is the crucial difference. Your perception is everything.

If you find yourself becoming sick too often, then there is likely either an immune system or other organic dysfunction which requires further investigation with a healthcare professional, or you may need to detoxify.

Instead of focusing on removing the symptoms, ask yourself why you became ill in the first place and restructure your life to remove that stressor. This will help you get well because your immune system can stop dealing with the cause of the illness and concentrate on removing the symptoms and effects already created. This is often called detoxification.

You can detoxify your body in a number of ways:

- **Nutritional detox**

You can start gently by simply removing the more obvious unhealthy foods in your diet or you can take a more intensive detox programme through fasting or liver or colon cleansing. Consider your current health and how long you have been toxifying your body, as well as what feels the most comfortable for you. Your naturopath can assist you in selecting the most effective option for your individual condition.

- **Environmental detox**

Pesticides and many household cleaning products contain chemicals which are absorbed through the skin and lungs and can be detrimental to your health. If you are overusing these products, reducing or eliminating exposure is advisable. Heavy metals can be detoxed with the help of a homeopath.

- **Emotional detox**

Anger and resentment can have a profound effect on the digestion system, immune system, perceptions, and general health. If you are harbouring such feelings toward significant people in your life, the wisest thing you can do for yourself is to find a way to release them through communication, apology or forgiveness.

- **Social detox**

Sometimes, certain people create more stress in our lives than they're worth. This is sometimes known as a "toxic relationship" and, if difficulties can't be resolved, then it may be time to thank them for their contribution to your life and let them go. If you choose to lose the friend or loved one; don't lose the lesson.

- **Electromagnetic detox**

Things like mobile phones, computers and high-definition televisions emit EMF and EMR which can cause stress within your body. Try to limit your exposure by using these items less. Of course, in our modern society it is difficult, if not impossible, to avoid them entirely, but you can help your body adapt to these stressors. By boosting your immune system and managing your emotions better, you change your ability to handle all forms of stress.

- **Heavy Metal Detox**

you can ask your homeopath and naturopath about this. Heavy metals can be found in things you ingest, inject or the air you breathe.

Change of Perception #5: You Don't Have to Know Something to *Know* It

We've talked about retraining yourself to see both sides, and that is important, but even when you don't *perceive* both sides of the whole picture with your conscious mind or senses, a part of you can *know* it. We are more than we think we are, and you don't always need to have the whole story to be able to "get the picture".

Look at the below for example.

Can You Read the Following?

fi yuo cna raed tihs, yuo hvae a sgtrane mnid too.

i cdnuolt blveiee taht I cluod aulaclty uesdnatnrd waht I was rdanieg. Aoccdrnig to a rscheearch at Cmabrigde Uinervtisy, it dseno't mtaetr in waht oerdr the ltteres in a wrod are, the olny iproamtnt tihng is taht the frsit and lsat ltteer be in the rghit pclae. The rset can be a taotl mses and you can sitll raed it whotuit a pboerlm. Tihs is bcuseae the huamn mnid deos not raed ervey lteter by istlef, but the wrod as a wlohe. Azanmig huh? yaeh and I awlyas tghuhot slpeling was ipmorantt!

When you let yourself go and stopped trying to focus on each letter or word, did you find that your understanding flowed more easily and your reading speed increased? If not, try it again. In most circumstances you are actually aware of the whole truth, but trying to limit your knowing by screening it through your perceptions can actually make you forget what you already intuitively "know".

When you don't trust yourself, and have actually been trained *not* to, you are much more likely to hand over responsibility to self-proclaimed "experts" and let them dictate your health choices. But the truth is that without relying on or deferring to any outside authority, you can still get the whole story. So, paradoxically, sometimes the greatest learning of all is *un*learning what we think we already know.

It's not that we don't know so much, but rather that we know so much that isn't so!

Paul Dirac

So it seems that a lot of what we have believed to be true may not be so – much of it could be either an unbalanced perception or an outright lie. That's a pretty challenging thought, isn't it? But it's still a matter of perception, and you can choose to see this as either a devastating revelation or a liberation, which is what it truly is. The truth is not missing, it's just more than what we thought it was.

The truth is what you make of it, and sometimes, like that elderly frightened woman, we make it negative and disempowering when, with a little thought, we could expand our vision and have an entirely different reality, a different story if you will. A woman can look into a mirror and focus only on her faults, ignoring her beautiful hair or skin or the light in her eyes, while a man can look into the same mirror, ignore the lines and beer belly, and see the young stallion he was at 25 years of age. Of course, the roles can be reversed, but the point is that you can create your own reality with your perceptions. Change your story and you change your life, balance your thoughts and the world comes into balance around you.

Some thoughts are lies, they are stories you made up.

Change Your Story!

If only one thing really rings true for you from this chapter, let it be the understanding that the happiness we have been searching for comes not from one-sided illusions, but from *balance*. We're all looking for fulfilment, but a life filled with nothing but elated happiness (even if it were possible, which it's not) is only half of life, it is "half-filment". And likewise, a life of sadness alone would also be only half-filment. Fulfilment comes when you embrace both sides of life and find the value in the highs *and* the lows. And surprisingly, when you can do this your highs won't be so high, your lows won't be so low, and you will lead a more balanced, loving and healthy life.

Faced with the choice between changing one's mind and proving there is no need to do so, almost everyone gets busy on the proof.

John Kenneth Galbraith

Top 7 Things to Create Love, Fulfillment & Health

1. **Have gratitude.** Be thankful for everything in your life. Keep a journal of all your blessings. It is only when you are grateful for what you've already been given that the universe will reward you with more.

2. **Change your environment.** If you surround yourself with negativity like dead plants or clutter, then you will attract chaos and ill health because what you see around you is decay. If you fill your life with living plants, fresh flowers, light and air through open windows, and clean spaces, you spontaneously attract more life, because that's what you're thinking about.

3. **Cut out visual and noise pollution.** Minimise your exposure to depressing images in newspapers, social media, television and movies. When listening to the radio, turn down the volume during advertisements. Read inspiring books and listen to beautiful music.

4. **Associate with those who you resonate with.** Be more selective about who you allow into your life. Choose people who support your efforts to evolve, or educate your existing friends to join you in your pursuit of what you want to be or do.

5. **Do what you love and love what you do.** What inspires you? What makes your soul sing? Do more of it. If you think you don't know what that is, then your challenge is to find it. You already know the answer deep inside, just have the courage to admit it to yourself. The next step is to find a way to earn a living from it, because when you can serve the world by doing what you're truly here for, you are living your truth and the sky is the limit.

6. **Relax.** Do less. Breathe deeper, go slower. Turn off the tech and phones occasionally and just *be*. If you give to yourself, then you'll have more to give to others. When you're rejuvenated, then give back, pay it forward. Surprise a stranger (and yourself) by doing something nice for them.

7. **Balance.** Love yourself by having a more balanced perspective about your life. Look for the other side of the coin and accept more. You can't always control what happens to you, but you can control what you make of it.

Changing beliefs is how we grow. Yesterday's unshakeable belief is today's amusing opinion, and today's medical certainty becomes tomorrow's primitive ignorance. Once-respected medical practices such as the use of lead, the removal of tonsils, and the opening of veins to release "bad blood" are now seen as harmful or ridiculous, and future doctors may look at the present-day reliance on drugs and surgery much as today's doctors regard the use of leeches in the past.

In medicine, as in all branches of knowledge, the more we learn, the more we realise there is still much to know, and that process never stops. An open mind never stops growing, and we are limited only by our will and our imagination.

With practice you can learn to see through the illusions that govern so much of our lives, and we hope we've given you a glimpse behind the illusion of illness and symptoms that you won't forget, and will continue to build upon. You have the rest of your life to work on expressing your true health potential, so asking more questions and challenging long-held socialised beliefs may be your best strategy for improving your health and wellness.

Health happens by choice, not by chance.

Andi Lew

References

Ewen, S., PR!: A Social History of Spin, Harper Collins.

Stauber & Rampton, Trust Us, We're Experts, Tarcher/Putnam 2001.

Robbins, J., Reclaiming Our Health, Kramer 1996.

Stay Connected

Chiropractic

Australian Chiropractor's Association
www.chiro.org.au

Other chiropractic websites
www.chiropractors.asn.au
www.worldchiropracticalliance.org

Integrative Care

Health Space Clinics
www.healthspaceclinics.com.au

Waters Co Filtration Australia
www.waterscoaustralia.com.au

Well Aware App for early detection
www.wellaware.life

Shopping

Therapeutic Pillow
www.the-pillow.com.au
Slim Secrets
www.slimsecrets.com.au
Beauty Food
www.beautyfood.com.au

Other Useful Websites

www.drmercola.com
www.additivealert.com.au
www.zacbushmd.com

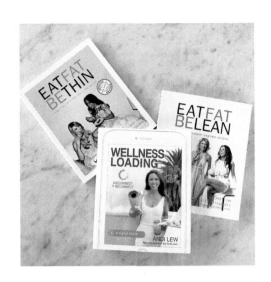

Other Books by Andi

Real Fit Food
The Modern Day Mother
Eat Fat Be Lean
Eat Fat Be Thin
Wellness Loading
#instalovers

BUY NOW!

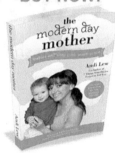

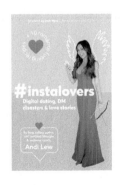

"Strong evidence-based, it's beautifully supportive".
Pinky McKay, Lactation Consultant & bestselling author

"Such a gentle, lovely way of giving advice. It's the charm of the book".
Suzanne Male, journalist & author

"Andi presents Attachment Parenting in an easy-to-understand way".
Dr Bill Sears, bestselling author

www.andilew.com
Follow Andi on Instagram @andi.lew

PROUD PARTNERS
of

Connected

a paradigm shift in how we view health

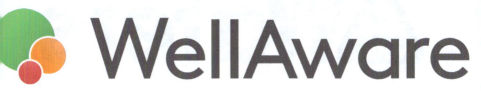

Imagine if the power for our health was made possible with a personalised, proactive tool that curbs risk factors before they lead to illness or even death. Imagine technology that saves and enhances the quality of our lives.

WellAware is an Australian owned, world first digital health technology developed for individuals and organisations to improve the mental, physical and emotional health of all Australians.

Powered by health data, we are backed by science and guided by Australia's health experts to focus on Mental Health, Heart, Type 2 Diabetes, Stroke, the 18 main Cancers as well as nutrition, sleep, exercise, anxiety and stress.

WellAware is the App that provides the tools and data needed to be in control of, transform and optimise your health for the rest of your life.

Our goal is to empower individuals to proactively look after their health and support the growing army of organisations seeking to advance the health of their teams, reduce risk and create a true culture of care.

WellAware is your health in your hands.

www.wellaware.life

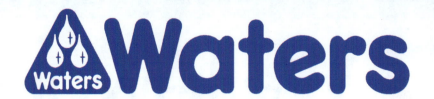

Our partners Waters Co Australia are a company with a priority to produce exceptionally high quality water filter systems, which turn contaminated tap water into great tasting, clean, fresh, alkaline, magnetised, and energised (live) mineral water. The products are made available to you at a sensible and affordable price with an environmental goal of providing a healthier and more sustainable option to disposable bottled water. By doing so we can lessen the impact associated with bottled water on our planet's precious resources, landfill and littering of our land, rivers and oceans.

The bonus is that whilst you're getting healthier, you're also looking after the health of our planet.

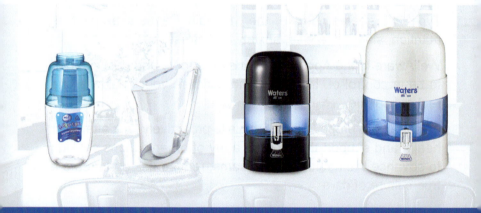

We are all connected.

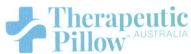

Therapeutic Pillow™ AUSTRALIA

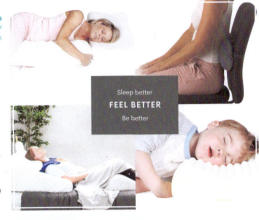

Sleep better
FEEL BETTER
Be better

Imagine sleeping and feeling better.

It's our mission to help every Australian enjoy a more restful, comfortable, and pain-free sleep – one pillow at a time!

We spend a third of our lives sleeping. Invest in quality, clinically designed pillows and support products that support your body day and night. Find the comfort you are looking for with our range of maternity pillows, sleeping pillows, back and neck supports, post-surgery supports, seniors comfort products, children pillows and mattress overlays to make you feel and sleep better.

Enjoy your best night sleep yet with latex and memory foam pillows trusted by Australian health professionals! the-pillow.com.au

Slim Secrets who are a healthy alternative to snacks to help you stay on track with your health and fitness goals. Sophie Monk created this new indulgence which is our delicious chocolatey treat. The keto friendly Protein Choc Fudge Brownie ticks so many boxes. It's gluten free and low in carbs, but best of all it has no sugar added so it helps keep sugar levels stable and may be suitable for some diabetics.

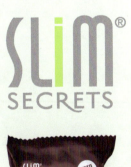

It contains collagen for an added boost to your beauty regime which can help support healthy hair, skin and nails.

Australian made Slim Secrets Choc Brownie is high in protein and a perfect pre or post workout snack. It can be eaten as is, or for some extra fun, you can warm it up a little and top it with yoghurt, berries or nuts and seeds.

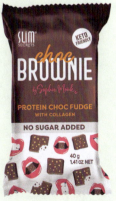